OBSTETRICS AND GYNECOLOGY ADVANCES

MENORRHAGIA AND DYSMENORRHEA

RISK FACTORS, DIAGNOSIS AND MANAGEMENT

OBSTETRICS AND GYNECOLOGY ADVANCES

Additional books in this series can be found on Nova's website under the Series tab.

Additional e-books in this series can be found on Nova's website under the e-book tab.

OBSTETRICS AND GYNECOLOGY ADVANCES

MENORRHAGIA AND DYSMENORRHEA

RISK FACTORS, DIAGNOSIS AND MANAGEMENT

TIMOTHY M. WELCH
EDITOR

New York

NOTICE TO THE READER

Library of Congress Cataloging-in-Publication Data

ISBN: 978-1-63482-552-8
Library of Congress Control Number: 2015936108

Published by Nova Science Publishers, Inc. † New York

Contents

Preface

Menorrhagia is defined as heavy menstrual loss. Its main determinant of management is the impact of menorrhagia on the woman's quality of life. This book examines the history of menorrhagia, which should elucidate the temporal aspects of the heavy menstrual blood loss and may shed light on the etiology of menorrhagia. The authors further provide instructions on how to examine and treat women with menorrhagia. Furthermore, the book outlines a diagnostic approach and concentrates on different therapies like combined oral contraceptive pills in contrast with surgical management. With an effective treatment management, it is possible to better achieve the diagnostics of heavy menstrual bleeding (HMB) although areas that need further research are highlighted. The clinical use of NF-kappaB (NF-kB) inhibitors, which play an important role in the regulation of the amount of menstrual bleeding and pain are also explored. In addition to menorrhagia, the authors of this book examine dysmenorrhea, pain associated with menstruation. It is also the most prevalent symptom in women with the painful condition of endometriosis. Ilaria Erasmo and Simone Ferrero examine the types of therapy for endometriosis-related dysmenorrhea and the various hormonal treatments shown to effectively and safely relieve pain, which they argue should be based on the preference of the patients, on the incidence of adverse effects and on the costs of treatment.

Chapter I – The objective definition of menorrhagia is heavy menstrual loss of greater than 80ml per menstrual cycle on consecutive menstruations. This quantification of menstrual loss is however not utilized in clinical practice because the main determinant of management is the impact of menorrhagia on the woman's quality of life. A significant source of anxiety surrounding the symptom of menorrhagia is the presence of serious pathology such as malignancy. Apprehension also arises due to the significant impact of menorrhagia on the physical, social, financial and emotional quality of life. A detailed history should elucidate the temporal aspects of the heavy menstrual blood loss and may shed light on the etiology of the menorrhagia. From the general history besides assessing the impact on the quality of life, the psychological background involving stress or eating disorders causing anovulatory heavy menses may be discerned. The history may also outline possible causes of menorrhagia such as relevant drug history including aspirin or warfarin and familial blood dyscrazias, the most common being von Willebrand's Disease. A gynaecological history of dysmenorrhoea and ovulatory pain may indicate the presence of endometriosis and adenomyosis, whereas postcoital bleeding may suggest cervical pathology. On general examination the degree of anaemia or the clinical features of hypothyroidism may come into focus. Gynaecological examination will assess the pelvic cavity to exclude the presence of palpable fibroids, ovarian tumours or lesions in the genital region. The history and examination will direct the relevant investigations that need to be employed. A complete blood count will assess the degree of anaemia and the blood indices such as the platelet count and mean corpuscular haemoglobin concentration. If indicated hormonal assessments may involve thyroid function tests and the determination of the presence of hyperprolactaemia leading to anovulatory menorrhagia. Imaging of the pelvic organs usually involves ultrasonic investigation performed both abdominally or transvaginally. More in-depth imagery with hysteroscopic visualization and biopsy of the endometrium is the gold standard to exclude intrauterine or submucosal pathology leading to menorrhagia. If the endometrium appears benign on hysteroscopic examination, in selected cases it may be appropriate to insert the levonorgestrel intrauterine system so as to enact a one-stop shop management of menorrhagia. Once malignancy has been excluded the treatment of menorrhagia initiates with conservative management leading to a spectrum of surgical interventions. Around one fifth of women once reassured that no serious pathology is evident will opt not to have treatment. Medical treatments such as nonsteroidal inflammatory agents, tranexamic acid and ethamsylate have been useful in stemming heavy menstrual loss. If appropriate and if the woman requires contraception, the oral contraceptive pill may be also used to treat menorrhagia. The levonorgestrel intrauterine device together with other treatments has been proposed as a first line treatment of menorrhagia. It is crucial for the success of the levonorgestrel intrauterine system that adequate counselling and reassurance of post insertion side-effects such as irregular vaginal bleeding are dealt with so as ensure patient compliance. Short-term medical treatment of severe menorrhagia is available. These include oral progestins norethisterone acetate and injectable progesterone, gonadotrophin releasing hormone analogues and selected progesterone receptor modulators. The latter are also useful in reducing uterine fibromyomatous volume. If the above measures do not succeed more invasive procedures may have to be employed. Treatments directly applied to the endometrium include transcervical resection of the endometrium, global endometrial ablative techniques such as the application of the thermal balloon, microwave or radiofrequency ablation of the endometrium. On occasion these locally ablative measures require repeat or further intervention. The last resort is hysterectomy which is the most invasive however the definitive treatment of menorrhagia.

Chapter II – The complaints of heavy menstrual bleeding (HMB) have a substantial impact on the gynecological services and in most of the cases, without any other disorders. Some treatment considerably improves the quality of life, being important to decide the assessment of the patients by providing the best treatment options. This guideline provides instructions on how to examine and treat women with menorrhagia. Despite this, symptoms can be extremely distressing and different treatments are currently available. The choice of treatment depends on symptoms as well as the known potential side effects and risks of medication. The present review outlines a diagnostic approach and concentrated on different medical therapies like combined oral contraceptive pills, oral progesterone and levonorgestrel-releasing intrauterine system in contrast with surgical management, like endometrial ablation, uterine artery embolization or hysterectomy. With an effective treatment management, it is possible to better achieve the diagnostics of HMB, although area for further research is highlighted.

Chapter III – Menstruation is an inflammatory process initiated by progesterone withdrawal, which elicits activation of the N-Kappa.b pathway. This triggers a complex inflammatory cascade involving the transcription of several genes coding for enzymes and inflammatory cytokines. Among the essential enzymes involved in this pathway are the cyclooxygenase enzymes, responsible for the synthesis of several prostaglandins, which play a pivotal role in the mechanism of menstrual bleeding and pain.

Chapter IV – Dysmenorrhea is the most symptoms in women with endometriosis; its intensity is often severe and causes a significant decrease in quality of life. It is often associated with other pain symptoms (such as deep dyspareunia, dyschezia, non-menstrual pelvic pain). The pathogenesis of dysmenorrhea in women with endometriosis remains uncertain; it may be due to nociceptive, inflammatory and neuropathic mechanisms. Two types of therapy for endometriosis-related dysmenorrhea are available:

pharmacological therapies that inhibit the growth of the endometriotic implants and surgical therapies, which aim to remove the endometriotic implants. Various hormonal treatments have been shown to effectively and safely relieve pain: non-steroidal anti-inflammatory drugs, progestins, androgens, combined oral contraceptive pill, gonadotropin releasing hormones analogues, gonadotropin releasing hormones antagonists and aromatase inhibitors. Hormonal therapies do not cure endometriosis, therefore patients require a long-term treatment. All hormonal therapies are contraceptive and, therefore, they cannot be administered to patients desiring to conceive. Given this background, the choice of the drug should be based on the preference of the patients, on the incidence of adverse effects and on costs. Surgical excision of endometriosis is a valuable option in patients with severe dysmenorrhea desiring to conceive, in those who have persistence of the symptom despite the administration of hormonal therapies and in those who have contraindications to the use of hormonal therapies. However, dysmenorrhea may recur after surgery if patients do not receive a post-operative hormonal therapy.

In: Menorrhagia and Dysmenorrhea
Editor: Timothy M. Welch
ISBN: 978-1-63482-552-8

Chapter I

Menorrhagia: Risk Factors, Diagnosis and Treatment

Yves Muscat Baron
Academic Department of Obstetrics and Gynaecology,
University of Malta Medical School, Malta

Abstract

The objective definition of menorrhagia is heavy menstrual loss of greater than 80ml per menstrual cycle on consecutive menstruations. This quantification of menstrual loss is however not utilized in clinical practice because the main determinant of management is the impact of menorrhagia on the woman's quality of life. A significant source of anxiety surrounding the symptom of menorrhagia is the presence of serious pathology such as malignancy. Apprehension also arises due to the significant impact of menorrhagia on the physical, social, financial and emotional quality of life.

A detailed history should elucidate the temporal aspects of the heavy menstrual blood loss and may shed light on the etiology of the menorrhagia. From the general history besides assessing the impact on the quality of life, the psychological background involving stress or eating disorders causing anovulatory heavy menses may be discerned. The history may also outline possible causes of menorrhagia such as relevant drug history including aspirin or warfarin and familial blood dyscrazias, the most common being von Willebrand's Disease. A gynaecological history of dysmenorrhoea and ovulatory pain may indicate the presence of endometriosis and adenomyosis, whereas postcoital bleeding may suggest cervical pathology. On general examination the degree of anaemia or the clinical features of hypothyroidism may come into focus. Gynaecological examination will assess the pelvic cavity to exclude the presence of palpable fibroids, ovarian tumours or lesions in the genital region.

The history and examination will direct the relevant investigations that need to be employed. A complete blood count will assess the degree of anaemia and the blood indices such as the platelet count and mean corpuscular haemoglobin concentration. If indicated hormonal assessments may involve thyroid function tests and the determination of the presence of hyperprolactaemia leading to anovulatory menorrhagia.

Imaging of the pelvic organs usually involves ultrasonic investigation performed both abdominally or transvaginally. More in-depth imagery with hysteroscopic visualization and biopsy of the endometrium is the gold standard to exclude intrauterine or submucosal pathology leading to menorrhagia. If the endometrium appears benign on hysteroscopic examination, in selected cases it may be appropriate to insert the levonorgestrel intrauterine system so as to enact a one-stop shop management of menorrhagia.

Once malignancy has been excluded the treatment of menorrhagia initiates with conservative management leading to a spectrum of surgical interventions. Around one fifth of women once reassured that no serious pathology is evident will opt not to have treatment. Medical treatments such as nonsteroidal inflammatory agents, tranexamic acid and ethamsylate have been useful in stemming heavy menstrual loss. If appropriate and if the woman requires contraception, the oral contraceptive pill may be also used to treat menorrhagia.

The levonorgestrel intrauterine device together with other treatments has been proposed as a first line treatment of menorrhagia. It is crucial for the success of the levonorgestrel intrauterine system that adequate counselling and reassurance of post insertion side-effects such as irregular vaginal bleeding are dealt with so as ensure patient compliance.

Short-term medical treatment of severe menorrhagia is available. These include oral progestins norethisterone acetate and injectable progesterone, gonadotrophin releasing hormone analogues and selected progesterone receptor modulators. The latter are also useful in reducing uterine fibromyomatous volume.

If the above measures do not succeed more invasive procedures may have to be employed. Treatments directly applied to the endometrium include transcervical resection of the endometrium, global endometrial ablative techniques such as the application of the thermal balloon, microwave or radiofrequency ablation of the endometrium. On occasion these locally ablative measures require repeat or further intervention. The last resort is hysterectomy which is the most invasive however the definitive treatment of menorrhagia.

Introduction

The term menorrhagia is the shorter version of menometrorrhagia. The Latin etymological derivation comes from meno for month, metra meaning womb and rhegynai to burst forth. Ancient Greek theories of menstruation emanating from Hippocrates and Aristotle perceived menorrhagia as a common event. In a population that was undernourished almost anorexic, this perception is paradoxic as lower body mass index is more likely to lead to oligoamenorrhoea rather than menorrhagia. These theories possibly stemmed from the cultural background of the time that made certain erroneous assumptions about the female body, resulting in a distortion of observations and their interpretation (Dean-Jones, 1989).

A number of theories have also been proposed regarding the physiological significance of menstruation from the time of Aristotle to the present in conjunction with the evolutionary changes in the uterus. The most recent theories on the evolution of menstruation include that menstruation evolved to cleanse the uterus of pathogens introduced by sperm, and the second suggests that the function of endometrial regression is to save energy by getting rid of tissue, rather than maintaining it in the absence of a viable pregnancy. Alternatively frequent or heavy menstruation is a reflection of infertility and a possible attraction to predation augmenting the evolutionary disadvantage with the application of natural selection. This concept has not yet been shown in comparative evolutionary models as in menstruating primates. Menstruation may also be a default situation in the absence of a pregnancy which is the most pressing aspect of evolution (Finn, 1989).

Menstruation was a very rare occurrence in the past. In the absence of contraception and the need to produce as many offspring as possible followed by a prolonged period of breastfeeding induced amenorrhoea and consequently the occurrence of regular menstruation was a rare event. The occurrence of menorrhagia was an even rarer event.

Accordingly menstruation in the evolutionary sense may be considered a negative factor in the course of evolution. Furthermore, most primitive animals were amenorrhoeic or would have menstruated infrequently, and many may have reproduced or passed away without ever having offspring (Finn, 1996).

Definition of Menorrhagia and Its Epidemiology

The objective definition of menorrhagia was determined from population studies whereby a threshold volume of 80ml of blood was lost in 10% of menstruating women. On average the amount of blood loss per menstruation without clots was estimated from these population studies as 35-50ml (Hallberg et al., 1966).

The above mentioned population studies utilized the alkaline haematin technique to quantify menstrual blood loss as implemented by Hallberg et al., in 1964. The alkaline haematin technique method involves the extraction of haem from used sanitary towels by applying 5% sodium hydroxide. Although alkaline haematin technique is considered to be the standard technique for estimating blood loss during menses, this method is costly, cumbersome and may be unacceptable to a significant proportion of women. For these reasons the alkaline haematin technique is usually applied in the research setting and not usually employed in clinical practice.

The main determinant of the clinical management of menorrhagia is its impact on the woman's quality of life. There appears to be a significant discordance ranging from 38 - 76% between women's self reporting of menstrual loss and the actual objective blood loss (Chimbira et al., 1980, van Eijkeren et al., 1986, Rybo, 1966).

This discordancy between actual quantification of menstrual loss and women's perception of blood loss has determined an alteration in the clinical definition of menorrhagia. According to the NICE guidelines the definition of menorrhagia has been modified as *"Excessive menstrual blood loss which interferes with a woman's physical, emotional, social and material quality of life and which can occur alone or in combination with other symptoms"* (NICE Guidelines, 2007). Menorrhagia has been shown to affect women's quality of life in a negative manner. Sule et al., (2013) have demonstrated all eight subdimensions of the SF-36 Quality of Life Scale including pain, general health, vitality, social role functioning, emotional functioning, and mental health are negatively effected by menorrhagia (Sule et al., 2013).

Tanaka et al., 2013 report increasing severity of menstrual symptoms including self-reported heavy bleeding resulted in more outpatient consultations and substantial absence from work. The estimated annual economic burden is substantial and was calculated to amount to 683 billion Japanese Yen (JPY) or approximately 8.6 billion United States Dollars (USD) (Tanaka et al., 2013). In general, heavy menstrual bleeding is associated with negative perceptions and limited social and professional activity, although all areas are significantly more affected in women experiencing heavy menstrual bleeding than normal menstrual bleeding.

Epidemiological studies indicate that menorrhagia affects varying proportions of women ranging from 8% to 27% of females in the reproductive age. The perception of heavy menstrual loss is also influenced by geographic location and the cultural background. When the sample studied is limited to older women the prevalence of heavy menstrual blood loss increases. In developing countries, the incidence of abnormal uterine bleeding affects about 5–15% of women of reproductive age whereas in developed countries the rates may be as high as 30% (Harlow and Campbell, 2003).

A Swedish study in 2014 found that 32% of women experienced heavy menstrual bleeding, 39% normal menstrual blood loss, 15% light menstrual blood loss and 14% no menstruation (Karlsson et al., 2014). In a Japanese study of 19,254 menstrual women 74% suffered from menstrual symptoms. A total of 50% reported dysmenorrhoea and 19% reported heavy bleeding. In a study on African American women 38.9% of women interviewed reported consulting a clinician for heavy menstrual loss and 46.1% believed that there no treatment could prevent it from occurring (Marsh et al., 2014). Menorrhagia is the main presenting problem in at least 50-70% of women requiring hysterectomy in the U.K. and USA (El-Hemaidi et al., 2007).

Anamnestic Features of Menorrhagia

A detailed anamnesis should elucidate the temporal aspects of the heavy menstrual blood loss and may shed light on the etiology of this symptom. The average duration of menstrual loss is usually defined as 7 days and the interval between cycles is 21 to 35 days. Rybo et al., (1966) indicated that 78% of the total menstrual loss occurred by the second day and 91% by the third day of menses while Haynes et al., (1977) reported that women with menorrhagia tended to have an increased loss in the first three days of menstruation. Recent literature has shown that approximately 4–8% of women report having menstrual periods longer than 7–8 days (Sioban and Campbell, 2003).

The pattern of bleeding may indicate the underlying pathology leading to menorrhagia. Intracyclical heavy bleeding is more likely to be due to endometrial polyps. Endometrial polyps cause greater intracyclical bleeding due to increased polyp metalloproteinases and cyclo-oxygenase production (Erdemoglu et al., 2008). Furthermore endometrial polyps have been noted to have increased microvascular density (Tokyol et al., 2009).

On the other hand extracyclical bleeding may be due to para-endometrial causes. The most common cause for para-endometrial menorrhagia are leiomyomas leading to the development of venule ectasia. Venule ectasia is thought to result from tumour and/or hypoxia-derived angiogenic factors and increased expression of oestrogen receptor causing spiral artery vasodilation (Fraser et al., 2007). A history of irregular menstruation associated with anovulation may suggest polycystic ovarian syndrome and possibly underlying endometrial hyperplasia and adenocarcinoma (Sweet et al., 2012).

During the consultation the woman may complain of fatigue and lethargy due to iron deficiency anaemia impacting the quality of life. Dysphagia and the occurrence of increased frequency of infection may due to altered immune response resulting from iron deficiency anaemia (Palacios S, 2011).

From the history the psychological background and personality of the woman may be discerned. In a Canadian study psychological disorders were diagnosed in 82.6% of women with functional uterine bleeding (Dutton 1965). A study in primary care demonstrated that women with psychological disorders were more likely than community controls to complain of heavy menstrual loss (odds ratio [OR] = 2.86, 95% confidence interval [CI] = 1.53-5.35) and heavy menses interfering with quality of life (OR = 3.69, 95% CI = 2.02-6.75) (Shapley et al., 2001). A study from the same authors indicated that women with psychological disturbance at the baseline consultation were more likely to present with menorrhagia six months later than women without distress (adjusted odds ratio 1.87, 95% CI 1.15, 3.02). Women with menorrhagia at baseline were less likely to develop psychological distress 6 months later than women with normal menses (adjusted odds ratio 1.09, 95% CI 0.73, 1.63) (Shapley et al., 2003). A significant source of anxiety surrounding the symptom of menorrhagia is the suspicion of the presence of serious pathology such as malignancy.

In cases of eating disorders leading to anovulatory heavy menstrual loss the patient or family may seek gynecological consultation before the diagnosis of primary psychiatric disturbance has been made. However the degree of psychiatric disorder and body weight in such patients may determine whether they do present with anovulatory heavy menstrual loss (Slupik, 1999).

The drug history may outline possible causes of menorrhagia such as relevant medications including aspirin or warfarin. Oral anticoagulation is associated with increased bleeding complications. Paradoxically, infrequent aspirin users reported more heavy menses than frequent users (21% vs. 8%, P = 0.01, and 56% vs. 38%, P = 0.03, respectively) (Mauer et al., 2011). Forty-seven women on oral anti-coagulants completing a pictorial bleeding chart indicated that the mean duration of menstruation increased from 5 days before starting oral anticoagulation therapy to 7 days after the commencement of treatment. Thirty-one (66%) of the 47 women who completed the pictorial bleeding chart experienced flooding or clots during menstruation (Huq et al., 2011).

In a study of eighty-one adolescents females on warfarin, 24 (30%) were referred to gynaecology due to heavy periods resulting in nineteen of these patients requiring treatment for menorrhagia (Peake et al., 2011). A drug history of tamoxifen may shed light on both benign and malignant causes for menorrhagia related to this treatment. Abnormal uterine bleeding occurs in more than 50% of women taking tamoxifen and may be due to endometrial polyp formation and/or endometrial carcinoma (Bakkum-Gamez et al., 2012). In contrast there have been cases whereby tamoxifen was utilized to treat myometrial hypertrophy causing menorrhagia (Fraser, 1987).

From the family history hereditary blood dyscrazias, the most common being von Willebrand's Disease may also be sought out. Bleeding diatheses in females generally present as heavy menstrual bleeding commencing at menarche and are present in 10.7% of adolescents compared to 3.2% of controls (Dilley et al., 2001). Von Willebrand's disease is the most common blood dyscrazia leading to menorrhagia with a prevalence of 5–20% (Matchar, 2004).

The United States Haemophilia Treatment Centres demonstrated that the menorrhagia was the most common bleeding symptom (198/253; 78.3%). In this survey the most frequent diagnoses were type 1 von Willebrand's disease (195/319; 61.1%), von Willebrand's disease type unknown (49/319; 15.4%) and factor VIII deficiency (40/319; 12.5%) (Byams et al., 2011). Eighty-five percent of all adult females with von Willebrand disease report menorrhagia and 37% give a history of severe postpartum haemorrhage. von Willebrand disease is a common cause for hospital admission due to menorrhagia (Sanders et al., 2014).

In a study on young Turkish women (mean age 20.68±10.34 years) 20% of the patients complaining of menorrhagia were diagnosed has having a bleeding disorder. The blood dyscrazias diagnosed in this study included 3 women with von Willebrand disease, 2 patients with low von Willebrand antigen, 1 case of probable von Willebrand disease, 3 cases of Bernard-Soulier syndrome, 2 cases of Glanzmann's thrombasthenia, 2 cases of immune thrombocytopenic purpura, 1 case of congenital factor VII deficiency (Suar Çakı et al., 2013).

A gynaecological history of dysmenorrhoea and ovulatory pain may indicate the presence of endometriosis or adenomyosis. Endometriosis most commonly afflicts women in the second and third decade of reproductive life. Menorrhagia is one component of the classic symptom complex of endometriosis. Women with this condition may also complain of dysmenorrhoea, dyspareunia, menorrhagia and infertility. A history of infertility in a woman with menorrhagia may suggest endometriosis as it co-exists in 30% - 40% of infertility cases (Okeke et al., 2011). In the presence of dysmenorrhoea endometriosis is the most common cause of secondary dysmenorrheoa (Osayande and Mehulic, 2014). In a national case control study in the U.K. 73% of women with endometriosis complained of menorrhagia (OR 4.0 [95% CI: 3.5-4.5]) compared with only 20% controls (Ballard et al., 2008). The co-existence of menorrhagia and endometriosis has been ascertained through the common a role for cyclooxygenase enzymes and prostaglandins (Sales and Jabbour, 2003).

Menorrhagia, together with pelvic pain and dysmenorrhoea are typical symptoms of adenomyosis. Adenomyosis is a pathological gynaecological condition characterised by benign invasion of the endometrium into the myometrium. It is often misdiagnosed, or is not easily recognised (Valentini et al., 2011). Moreover, adenomyosis and uterine fibroids commonly coexist (80%) in the same uterus, and differentiating the contribution of each pathology may be difficult to extricate. Although adenomyosis has been recognized for over a century, reliable epidemiological studies on this condition are limited, because until now only postoperative diagnoses were possible (Taran et al., 2013).

In a study of 710 premenopausal patients undergoing hysterectomy with the histological finding of adenomyosis, dysmenorrhoea was the most common complaint, occurring in 81.7% of patients and co-existed most frequently with heavy menstruation. Increasing age and the severity of dysmenorrheoa in women with adenomyosis, were associated with the risk of heavy periods (Li et al., 2014). Although adenomyosis is a benign condition, a malignancy in the form of endometrioid adenocarcinoma is often associated with adenomyosis. This malignancy is frequently of early stage and low histological grade giving an excellent prognosis (Bergeron et al., 2006).

For a large proportion of women no cause for menorrhagia is diagnosed known as dysfunctional uterine bleeding. Dysfunctional uterine bleeding is therefore a diagnosis of exclusion (Fraser et al., 1994). From the age of the patient, idiopathic menorrhagia may be categorized as ovulatory or anovulatory. Ovulatory causes for idiopathic menorrhagia are more likely in the 20 - 40 age group, whereas anovulatory reasons for menorrhagia mainly occur at the extremes of reproductive life. Anovulatory bleeding usually results from inadequate progesterone levels. As a corollary this leads to reduced progesterone induced endometrial stromal cell tissue factor and plasminogen activator inhibitor-1 production. Low progesterone due to anovulation leads to increased matrix metalloproteinase activity and increased angiogenic factor expression. The combination of these effects on the various stromal, haemostatic and vascular factors results in vessel instability with diminished hemostasis, each cumulatively predisposing to menorrhagia (Lockwood, 2011).

A family history of idiopathic menorrhagia may also be elucidated from the anamnesis. In a study of 152 women with idiopathic menorrhagia compared to 56 healthy regularly menstruating women, a strong association was found between idiopathic menorrhagia and a family history of heavy menstrual bleeding (r=0.68) (Kuzmima et al., 2011). As discussed earlier the perception of blood loss may be influenced by the psychological and familial background.

Although the mechanisms underlying the causes of heavy menstrual blood loss remain to be elucidated, prostaglandins have been firmly implicated (Duckitt and Collins, 2012). Emerging evidence supports a role for cyclooxygenase enzymes, prostaglandins and prostaglandin receptor signaling pathways in the endometrium. These factors all influence the promotion of angiogenesis and vascular function (Jabbour et al., 2006).

Prostaglandin I synthase and the prostacyclin receptor were significantly expressed during the menstrual phase of the cycle compared with all other phases ($P < 0.05$) (Battersby et al., 2004). A significant elevation in expression of cyclooxygenase mRNA in endometrium was demonstrated in women with menorrhagia when compared with endometrium obtained from controls with normal menses. Tissue culture stimulated with prostaglandin E2 caused a significant elevation of prostaglandin metabolites when compared with normal menstruations (Smith et al., 2007).

Functional alterations in small myometrial arteries could contribute to idiopathic menorrhagia. The response of myometrial blood vessels in women with idiopathic menorrhagia was significantly different from women with normal menses when these vessels were exposed in vitro to various vasoactive agents such as endothelin-1 and N(w)-nitro-L arginine methyl ester and bradykinin. Vascular tension mimicking vasoconstriction was increased with the inhibition of cyclooxygenase-derived products ($P < 0.05$) (Mints et al., 2008).

Examination

On examination specific clinical manifestations suggesting iron deficiency anaemia may be demonstrable. These include pallor, fatigue, atrophic changes in the epithelium, oral lesions such as angular cheilosis, and koilonychia (Palacios, 2011).

Clinical manifestation of thyroid disease may be noted in women complaining of menorrhagia. Both hyperthyroidism and hyperthyroidism may lead to abnormal uterine bleeding. Both oligomenorrhoea and menorrhagia are the most common menstrual disturbances in hypothyroidism (Krassas et al., 1999). Cases of acute menorrhagia causing life-threatening anaemia that resulted from profound hypothyroidism have reported (Moragianni and Somkuti, 2007). The occurrence of menorrhagia and easy bruising may occur in patients with moderate to severe hypothyroidism sometimes linked to acquired von Willebrand's disease (Attivissimo et al., 1995).

Clinical manifestations of other endocrinopathies may also be causes of associated menorrhagia. Obesity, acne and hirsutism may be associated with polycystic ovary syndrome. A high body mass index or sudden weight loss may be related to uncontrolled diabetes mellitus. The elucidation of galactorrhoea linked with anovulation may indicate the presence of hyperprolactinemia.(Sweet et al., 2012).

Gynaecological examination will assess the pelvic cavity to exclude the presence of palpable fibroids, ovarian tumours or lesions in the genital region. Uterine myomas may be found on abdominal and pelvic examination. The mechanism of heavy menses is poorly understood however anecdotal evidence suggests that thin friable vessels in the presence of myomas or adenocarcinoma may lead to significant blood loss. The disturbed angiogenesis in these situations may be due to the unbalanced release of angiogenic factors from the tumours involved (Jones and Harris, 2011). Similarly polyps noted on speculum examination are associated with increased angiogenesis and abnormal vessel formation leading to heavy menstruation (Lockwood, 2011).

Speculum examination may also reveal endometriotic implants in the externally visible genital tract. Endometriosis can be located in the cervix and vagina, whereby digital examination will detect scarring and puckering especially in the posterior vaginal wall, which is closely related to the frequently affected rectovaginal septum. Endometriotic implants have been found in the perineal scars of previous episiotomies or in the Bartholin's gland (Acien and Velasco, 2013).

Speculum examination may reveal malignancy arising from the cervix or carcinomatous tissue may be seen issuing out of the cervix. In developing countries the majority of cases of cervical cancer are diagnosed at an advanced stage as cytology based screening programmes are ineffective. Visual inspection with Lugol's iodine and acetic acid have been compared with Papanicolaou smear, and colposcopic directed biopsy. In low resource settings, screening of carcinoma cervix by Pap smear can be replaced by cheaper and easily available visual methods like Lugol's iodine which has the high sensitivity to detect any grade of dysplasia, with a reasonable specificity (Ghosh et al., 2012).

Investigation

A complete blood count will reveal the degree of anaemia and the differential assessment may also point to specific diagnosis. The most common haematological aberration related to menorrhagia is microcytic hypochromic anaemia (Ali, 1976). Leucocytosis may arise in the presence of pelvic inflammatory disease resulting in heavy menstruation (Peiper and Soper, 1994).

Thrombocytosis is a common disorder in patients diagnosed with iron deficiency anaemia. The decreased platelet counts commonly found iron deficiency anaemia is rarely reported in clinical practice. The exact mechanism of the occurrence of thrombocytopenia in iron deficiency anaemia remains unclear (Ibrahim et al., 2012). The comprehensive haematological profile suggested are a complete blood count, peripheral smear, activated partial thromboplastin time, ristocetin cofactor assay, prothrombin time, factor VIII and fibrinogen assays must be performed (Suar Çakı et al., 2013).

Hormone function tests as part of investigating menorrhagia span gonadotrophins, sex steroids and thyroid function tests. A 3 to 1 luteinizing hormone: follicular stimulating hormone ratio and low luteal progesterone suggest polycystic ovarian syndrome. Hyperprolactaemia in isolation or in conjunction with polycystic ovarian syndrome may lead to anovulatory menstrual disorders.

Abnormal thyroid function tests mainly reveal elevated thyroid stimulating hormone diagnostic of hypothyroidism induced menorrhagia.

There is a suggestion that when the levels of thyroid hormones improved, a reduction in menorrhagia was noted. This menstrual improvement was accompanied by a significant decline in random serum thyroid-stimulating hormone levels and rise of thyroxine levels compared to those found in the group with a negative response to the thyrotropin-releasing hormone test (Wilansky and Greisman, 1989). There is a suggestion that the more appropriate thyroid function test in women with unexplained menorrhagia should involve thyrotrophin releasing hormone (Weeks, 2000).

Imaging

Initially abdominal ultrasound was utilized to correlate the sonographic appearance of the endometrium and histopathologic findings. Abnormally thick endometrium was associated with endometrial polyps formation, endometrial carcinoma, hyperplasia, and adenomyosis (Fleischer et al., 1986).

Abdominal ultrasound has been superceded by the transvaginal approach. In a Scandinavian study on 51 premenopausal women with abnormal vaginal bleeding there was good agreement between histology and transvaginal ultrasound. Utilizing a cut-off point of greater than or equal to 8 mm endometrial thickness the sensitivity in diagnosing endometrial pathology was 67% and the specificity 75% (Smith et al., 1991).

In the case of menorrhagia due to uterine myomas a transvaginal scan may categorize the size and anatomical relation of the myoma. This may differentiate between intracavitary myoma, submucous or myometrial fibroids. Myomas 3cm or less sited in the endometrial cavity or submucosally are amenable to hysteroscopic resection (Perrot et al., 2002).

In cases of adenomyosis the presence of heterotopic endometrial glands and stroma in the myometrium may be noted sonographically. Furthermore adjacent to adenomyosis, smooth muscle hyperplasia reveals itself on transvaginal scanning as cystic dilatation of heterotopic glands and heterogeneity of the myometrial echotexture. Another finding in adenomyosis is antero-posterior asymmetry of the uterus. Transvaginal ultrasound scanning of the uterus with adenomyosis has a sensitivity of 62 to 89% and a specificity of 89 to 96% (Perrot et al., 2002).

Endometrial polyps causing menorrhagia are best noted in the follicular stage when the hyperechoic polyp is well defined within the hypoechoic endometrial background. The diagnosis of endometrial polyps is more difficult in luteal phase. The application of Power Doppler may reveal the vasculature in the supporting central pedicle. For endometrial polyps transvaginal ultrasound scanning has a sensitivity of 75%. Contrast media in the endometrial cavity may be useful to diagnose polyps that are smaller than 3 mm (Perrot et al., 2002).

During the last decade the visualization of the endometrial cavity utilizing the hysteroscope has become the gold standard investigation for abnormal menstrual bleeding. There appears o be a general consensus that in most patients, the combination of transvaginal ultrasonography and endometrial biopsy with diagnostic hysteroscopy in the out-patient setting could replace the need for dilation and curettage. Hysteroscopy has been reported to have sensitivity of 94.2%, specificity of 88.8%, negative predictive value of 96.3% and positive predictive value of 83.1% in differentiating between normal or abnormal endometrial histopathology. The highest specificity of hysteroscopy was in detecting endometrial polyps, whereas the lowest diagnostic specificity was in diagnosing hyperplasia. The presence of focal lesions such as endometrial polyps is high in abnormal uterine bleeding strengthening the premise that the most beneficial approach is to proceed with hysteroscopy complemented by endometrial biopsy (Revel and Shushan, 2002).

There appears to be a theoretical concern that the application of distension media to flush the uterine cavity may lead to retrograde dissemination of endometrial pathology (Revel and Shushan, 2002). In a small, study assessing peritoneal washings following laparoscopic assisted vaginal hysterectomy and total abdominal hysterectomy 14 (10.3%) of the patients treated laparoscopically had positive peritoneal cytology compared to only 7 (2.8%) of the control population. The clinical significance of the dissemination of endometrial cells during hysteroscopy is still undetermined (Sonoda et al., 2001).

Miniaturization of hysteroscopes and ancillary instrumentation such as the development of bipolar intrauterine systems, has facilitated 'see and treat' outpatient hysteroscopy, so that it should no longer be considered simply an outpatient diagnostic modality (Clark, 2004).

The acceptability of these procedures by women has also to be taken in consideration. A study comparing three outpatient procedures as regards performance patient acceptability and cost effectiveness was carried out by Crithley et al., (2004). Minor adverse events including shock and patient distress occurred in 16% and 10% of women for hysteroscopy and biopsy procedures respectively. Adequate endometrial sampling was obtained in pipelle biopsy in 79% of moderate-risk women, but only 43% of high-risk women. In contrast the Tao brush was more successful than the Pipelle sampling in postmenopausal (high-risk) women (72%) and obtained results in moderate-risk women (77%). Ultrasound provided more visualizations than for hysteroscopy in both the low-risk and the moderate-risk group. Moreover ultrasound was significantly better than hysteroscopy at detecting fibroids, but hysteroscopy significantly better for polyps.

Resource utilization tended to be higher in the moderate- and low-risk women. Cost-effectiveness between investigation options in the high-risk group did not differ significantly with the option involving hysteroscopy being marginally better than ultrasound. About 60% of premenopausal women with abnormal bleeding reported that their symptoms were not 'much improved' at 10 months (Crithley et al., 2004).

The comparison of various investigative modalities of menorrhagia has been carried out to elucidate the most efficacious combination. In a multi-centre, randomized, controlled trial of four hundred women with abnormal uterine bleeding, the investigators found that transvaginal sonography combined with Pipelle endometrial biopsy and outpatient hysteroscopy was as effective as inpatient hysteroscopy and curettage. Transvaginal sonography was confirmed as a cost-effective, sensitive, and well-tolerated method to evaluate most women with abnormal bleeding (Davidson and Dubinsky, 2003).

Management

Women with menorrhagia frequently present in the acute stage with severe menstrual blood loss. This loss is rarely life-threatening and can be treated on an outpatient basis with oral medication. In young women wishing to have children tranexamic acid in the dose of one gram every eight hours should stem the blood loss. The dose of tranexamic acid can be titrated with the impact on blood loss the maximum dose allowed is 4 grams per day. Long-term treatment with tranexamic acid may result in disturbances in colour vision necessitating discontinuation of treatment. Caution must be applied when prescribing tranexamic acid in patients with a history or family history of thromboembolic disease.

Alternatively norethisterone acetate in doses ranging from 5 mg to 10 mg four times daily may also reduce blood loss in the acute stage (Lethaby et al., 2008). Prolonged treatment with norethisterone may lead to polycythaemia and impaired glucose tolerance. These measures will allow time so that the appropriate investigations may be carried out as outlined above. Moreover iron supplementation with ferrous sulphate will augment the haemoglobin content to reverse the transient anaemia that may have occurred may also attenuate the menorrhagia. The patient complaining of menorrhagia should be advised to rest and avoid any arduous work.

Most of the first line investigations outlined above aim at excluding malignancy. If malignancy has been diagnosed then the appropriate oncological referral has to be expedited. Through the various investigations to exclude malignancy the aetiology for the menorrhagia may also be diagnosed. In this manner endometrial pathology such as polyps, Mullerian anomalies and submucosal fibroids may be diagnosed. In such cases the treatment of choice is tailored to the pathology including excision of the polyps, uterine septum or the submucosal fibroids by hysteroscopic resection.

Submucosal fibroids larger than 3cm may be reduced in size by utilizing luteinizing hormone releasing hormone agonists such as goserelin hydrochloride 3.6 mg given for 3 to 6 months. Alternatively submucosal fibroids may be excised in part over two or more hysterocopic sessions. In all cases of resection of submucosal fibroids patients must be consented for heavy intraoperative loss that may need medication such as tranexamic acid, blood transfusion and as a last resort hysterectomy.

In cases of large fibroids associated with menorrhagia, myomectomy or arterial embolization may be employed. Hysterectomy is the definitive treatment for menorrhagia but is costly in terms of morbidity, loss of productivity, patient satisfaction and also in economic terms (Sweet, 2012).

Although no agent is currently approved for the shrinkage of large fibroids, emerging evidence suggests the potential for long-term medical management of uterine fibroids (Singh and Belland, 2015). Recent clinical trials have demonstrated the efficacy of ulipristal acetate in the medical management of leiomyomas (Donnez et al., 2015). Barlow et al., have shown that in comparison to menorrhagia in the placebo group, a large proportion of women treated with ulipristal acetate (63.1% of those on 5 mg/day and 71.3% of those on 10 mg/day) experienced rapid arrest of menstruation or oligoamenorrhoea as evidenced by pictorial blood loss assessment charting (Barlow et al., 2014). Alternatively ulipristal acetate may be utilized pre-operatively so as to make the leiomyoma more amenable to surgery. Donnez et al., have shown that a reduction of the order of 21% in total fibroid volume was achieved with ulipristal acetate (Donnez et al., 2012).

If malignancy or any other physical causes have been excluded during hysteroscopy, treatment in the form of insertion of the levonorgestrel intrauterine system (LNG-IUS) may be employed acting as one stop shop management (Muscat Baron et al., 2012). In this latter study it was noted that menorrhagia was satisfactorily treated with the LNG-IUS in 93.5% of patients which is one of the highest success rates of this treatment for menorrhagia reported in scientific literature (Muscat Baron et al., 2012).

Comparative trials suggest that use of the LNG-IUS may be considered as a effective therapeutic alternative to endometrial ablative techniques or hysterectomy in women complaining of heavy menstrual loss (Inki et al., 2006) (Hurskainen et al., 2006). Not only is the volume of blood loss reduced but also the cycle length is shortened with the application of the LNG-IUS (Luukainen, 2000).

The therapeutic effect is translated through the effect of the levonorgestrel intrauterine system on the endometrium inducing epithelial atrophy consequently resulting in diminished menstrual loss. Reduction of excessive blood loss may be seen as early as the first menstruation after insertion, and at 1 year the reduction is more than 90%. Eighty percent of women may go on to become amenorrhoeic after two years having applied the levonorgestrel intrauterine system.

The high success rate in this study (Muscat Baron et al., 2012) may be attributed to a number of variables. In this study correct placement of the intra-uterine system following the endometrial biopsy may have been ascertained especially in those cases where general anaesthesia was requested by the women. This reduced the risk of inappropriate application of the LNG-IUS. Furthermore this secure placement of the LNG-IUS decreased the risk of spontaneous expulsion which only occurred in 1 patient in this study. Spontaneous expulsion rates of the levonorgestrel intra-uterine system of up to 4.5 - 5.9% have been quoted in the literature (Jensen et al., 2008) (Guttinger et al., 2007).

Endometrial biopsy immediately prior the insertion of the levonorgestrel intrauterine system may also have contributed to the efficiency of the LNG-IUS in treating the heavy menstrual loss. Endometrial biopsy may have partially "denuded" the endometrium allowing direct application of the LNG-IUS reservoir releasing the levonorgestrel directly on to the endometrial basal layer inducing glandular atrophy (Muscat Baron et al., 2012).

As mentioned earlier 20% of young women with menorrhagia under the age of 35 years should be investigated for blood dyscrazias such as von Willebrand disease. The latter condition has been shown to respond to oral contraception. Treatment consists of combined hormonal contraceptives which presumably induce human endometrial stromal cell tumour factor and plasminogen activating factor 1 levels to compensate for the hemostatic defect attendant such patients (James et al., 2004).

Thyroid function tests may reveal hypothyroidism related to the menorrhagia. Replacement therapy with thyroxine has been shown to resolve menorrhagia within three to six months. Moreover follow-up from one to three years indicated that the menorrhagia did not recur while on thyroxine replacement therapy (Wilansky and Griesman, 1989). In conjunction with hypothyroidism there may also co-exist an acquired form of von Willebrand disease. Although the acquired form of von Willebrand disease is more frequently associated with lympho-myeloproliferative and cardiovascular disorders, it can also occur in solid tumors and in immunological disorders and hypothyroidism with a frequency of approximately 2 to 5%. Treatment with thyroxine replacement therapy will reverse the acquired form of von Willebrand disease (Federici et al., 2011).

A high body mass index if attenuated with dietary modification and calorie expending exercise may manage polycystic ovarian syndrome. In the presence of acne and hirsutism, menorrhagia due to polycystic ovary syndrome may also be effectively treated with the combined oral contraception. Oral contraception reverses endometrial thickness leading to a reduction in menses (Caserta et al., 2014). With co-existing dysmenorrhoea, menorrhagia can also be treated with non steroidal anti-inflammatory drugs. Caution must always be exercised when prescribing nonsteroidal anti-inflammatory agents in women with a past history of bronchial asthma and peptic ulceration (Sweet, 2012). A possible scheme at implementing treatment for heavy menstrual loss is depicted in Table I.

Medical Management of Heavy Menstrual Loss in the Acute and Long-Term

Over the past two decades if medical treatments fail, resort to direct treatment to the endometrium leading to its destruction has become more commonly implemented. Initially endometrial ablation was carried out by transcervical endometrial resection via hysteroscopy. More recent "second-generation" ablative techniques such as the thermal balloon, radiofrequency or microwave ablation offer day-case surgical resolution to menorrhagia. Treatment success of these "second-generation" ablative techniques is highly dependent on the complete destruction of the endometrium. Endometrial ablation is most effective if employed when endometrial thickness is less than four millimeters. Thin endometrial layers may be found in the immediate postmenstrual phase, which however is not always practical in the perspective of elective day surgery.

Pre-operative endometrial thinning may also be induced medically by utilizing hormonal agents. The most commonly evaluated hormonal agents are goserelin (gonadotrophin-releasing hormone analogue) and danazol. Research suggests that goserelin and danazol reduce operating time requiring less endometrium to be resected and improve safety by reducing absorption of glycine, the usual fluid used for intraoperative uterine cavity distension (Tan and Lethaby, 2013). Goserelin induced more consistent endometrial thinning than danazol, although both achieved satisfactory results. In the long-term the effect of these agents on longer-term postoperative outcomes decreased with time. In the case of "second-generation" ablative techniques no benefits of goserelin pre-operative treatment was apparent. Goserelin possesses the side effects related to a pseudo-menopause whereas andronization may occur with danazol (Tan and Lethaby, 2013).

Transcervical endometrial resection of the endometrium was the first minimally invasive surgical technique used to treat menorrhagia. The procedure requires a certain level of surgical expertise as perforation to the uterus and injury to the viscera may occur. Moreover fluid overload has its risks whereby intravasation of only one litre of glycine may lead to hyponatraemia equilavent to a decrease in 10 milliequivalents of serum sodium.

Patient satisfaction scores suggest that transcervical endometrial resection was similar to microwave endometrial ablation. One-hundred and eighty-nine women returned questionnaires (72%) after a minimum of 10 years post-treatment with either transcervical endometrial resection or microwave endometrial ablation. Satisfaction rates were similar 77/129 (60%) in the microwave cohort compared to 70/134 (52%) in the resection group. Even bleeding and pain scores were highly significantly diminished and similar following both transcervical endometrial resection or microwave endometrial ablation resulting in amenorrhoea rates of 88% and 83% respectively (Sambrook et al., 2009). However the hysterectomy rate after 10 years was significantly different with 22 (17%) in the microwave endometrial ablation group and 38 (28%) in the transcervical endometrial resection group (95% CI: -0.21, -0.13). The authors concluded that the surgical advantages, lower costs and fewer hysterectomies, indicated that microwave endometrial ablation was superior to transcervical endometrial resection for the surgical treatment for heavy menstrual loss (Sambrook et al., 2009).

Table I. Scheme outlining possible medical treatment of heavy menstrual loss in both the acute and long-term with and without of the gynaecological requirements

Medication	Acute Episode of Heavy Menstrual Loss	Long-term Heavy Menstrual Loss	Long-term Heavy Menstrual Loss with Contraception	Long-term Heavy Menstrual Loss with Dysmenorrhoea	Long-term Heavy Menstrual Loss with Contraception and Dysmenorrhoea
Oral Progestins (Norethisterone Acetate)	1st Line	Not recommended	Not recommended	Not recommended	Not recommended
Antifibrinolytics (Tranexamic Acid)	1st Line	1st Line	Not recommended	Not recommended	Not recommended
Levornorgestrel Intrauterine System	Not recommended	1st Line	1st Line	1st Line	1st Line
Nonsteroidal anti-inflammatory	Not recommended	2nd Line	Not recommended	1st Line	Not recommended
Combined Oral Contraceptive pill	Not recommended	2nd Line	1st Line	1st Line	1st Line
Progestin in Luteal phase	Not recommended	Not recommended	Not recommended	Not recommended	Not recommended

Comparison between transcervical endometrial resection and the second generation ablative techniques has revealed no difference in efficacy in treating menorrhagia or in patient satisfaction. However the level of surgical expertise required was much lower in the second generation ablative techniques. This translated in lower operating times a gain on average of 15 minutes (14.9, 95% CI 10.1 to 19.7). However in second generation ablative techniques local anaesthesia was more likely to be employed (RR 2.8, 95% CI 1.8 to 4.4) and equipment failure was more likely (RR 4.3, 95% CI 1.5 to 12) with second-generation ablation.

Complications following second generation ablative techniques were less likely than transcervical endometrial resection. Second generation ablative procedures were less likely to have fluid overload, uterine perforation, cervical lacerations and hematometra than women undergoing the more traditional type of ablation and resection techniques. Minor side-effects such as nausea, vomiting and uterine cramping were more commonly found in the second generation ablative techniques. Recurrence of menorrhagia requiring either further surgery of any kind or hysterectomy specifically was reduced with second-generation ablative methods compared to first-generation ablation up to 10 years after surgery but not at earlier follow up.

Endometrial ablation techniques offer a less invasive surgical alternative to hysterectomy. Most of the newer techniques are technically easier to perform than traditional hysteroscopy-based methods however equipment failures need to be addressed. Overall, the existing evidence suggests that success, satisfaction rates and complication profiles of newer techniques of endometrial ablation compare favourably with hysteroscopic techniques.

Apart from patient safety, the cost-effectiveness of any treatment modality of menorrhagia has to be included in the equation of clinical governance. Hysterectomy which until recently was the most common surgical treatment of menorrhagia is associated with high morbidity, reduced productivity and high health care costs. Global endometrial ablation such as NovSure® provides a surgical alternative with reduced morbidity, cost, and recovery time. A recent model analyses showed lower costs for NovaSure-treated women than for those treated with other global endometrial ablation modalities or hysterectomy over all time frames. Re-ablation with the NovSure® for recurrence of menorrhagia showed a 43%-71% reduction. Moreover there were 69%-88% fewer added interventions and complications for NovaSure-treated patients compared to other global endometrial ablation techniques. Another added benefit of this treatment involved fewer days lost from work and short-term morbidity (Miller et al., 2015).

When both medical and minimally invasive surgical techniques fail to treat menorrhagia resort to hysterectomy may have to be employed. Carey et al., (2014) have determined the pathologic findings in hysterectomy specimens after failed global endometrial ablation. The usual reasons for failed global endometrial ablation is the presence of adenomyosis and leiomyomas both of which frequently co-exist. The histology reports of these specimens showed uterine leiomyomas in 33 specimens (49%). Persistent menorrhagia occurred in the presence of intramural myomas 15(44%) of women. Another 42% underwent hysterectomy because of pain mainly associated with haematometra. Haematometra was a significant finding in women who underwent hysterectomy because of persistent pain after global endometrial ablative techniques. A possible pathologic predictor of global endometrial ablation failure may be intramural leiomyomas (Carey et al., 2014).

Another cause for failures of global endometrial ablation treatment is the presence of adenomyosis. Mengerink et al., (2014) have shown that of 213 patients who underwent NovaSure therapy, 22 (10.3%) required hysterectomy because heavy menstrual loss persisted post-operatively. Ten women (45%) of failed NovaSure treatment exhibited adenomyosis in their hysterectomy specimens. A control group of patients who underwent hysterectomy without prior treatment with NovaSure had similar prevalence of adenomyosis (74/173, 42.8%). Although incidences of adenomyosis in this study was similar in both arms, the NovaSure-failure group had a significantly higher prevalence of deep seated adenomyosis (>2,5mm endometrial penetration) (9/22, 40.9%) than the control group (37/173, 21.4%; $p<0,05$). This paper intimated that endometrial ablation may have induced deep seated adenomyosis (Mengerink et al., 2014).

Moderately sized fibroids can be removed by laparoscopic assisted hysterectomies in multiparous women. Uterine sizes of 12 centimetres equivalent to 16 weeks gestation (weight 800g) are amenable to this surgical treatment (Shiota et al., 2011). In the case of larger fibroid uteri, laparoscopic morcellation until recently was a common mode of treatment for large leiomyomas. However in cases of large fibroids, laparoscopic morcellation is bound to decrease in favour of hysterectomy due to the fear of spillage of malignant cells during laparoscopic morcellation (Della Badia and Karini, 2010).

Conclusion

Menorrhagia is a symptom which affects up to one third of women of reproductive age. This symptom requires careful assessment by a detailed history and examination in an effort to differentiate between a wide spectrum of aetiologies which may cause menorrhagia. The history and examination will direct the investigation and imaging techniques required to ascertain a diagnosis. Of overarching importance is the exclusion of the presence of malignancy. Non malignant causes for menorrhagia range from blood dyscrazias especially in young women, anatomical reasons such as endometrial polyps and leiomyomas and endocrinopathies including hypothyroidism, polycystic ovariuan syndrome and hyperprolactaemia. In a large proportion of women no cause can be found, classified as ovulatory or anovulatory idiopathic menorrhagia. Ovulatory causes for menorrhagia have been associated with prostaglandin function whereas anovulatory reasons are related to inadquate levels of progesterone.

Treatment of menorrhagia will then be tailored to the causes of this symptom. Once reassured a proportion of women will not require further treatment. Anatomical reasons may be treated during the investigation phase as in the case of hysteroscopic extirpation of endometrial polyps. Medical treatments range from anti-fibrinolytic agents, nonsteroidal anti-inflammatory drugs, and hormonal therapy. Hormonal therapy delivered directly to the endometrium in the form of the levonorgestrel intrauterine system has become first line treatment of menorrhagia.

If conservative management fails then minimal invasive surgical techniques may be employed. Transcervical endometrial resection is mainly reserved for leiomyomas impinging on the endometrial cavity. Medical treatment in the form of goserelin hydrochloride or ulipristal acetate may shrink leiomyomas making them more amenable to endometrial resection. Second generation ablative techniques such as the thermal balloon, microwave and radiofrequency ablation have largely replaced transcervical endometrial resection.

Despite all efforts to treat menorrhagia conservatively or by minimally invasive surgery resort to hysterectomy may still be required. In cases of moderately sized uteri laparoscopic assisted vaginal hysterectomy may be employed to treat the heavy menstrual loss. Hysterectomy may be implemented in large leiomyomatous uteri and will then be the denifitive treatment of fibroid related menorrhagia.

References

Acién, P; Velasco, I. Endometriosis: A Disease That Remains Enigmatic. *ISRN Obstet Gynecol.*, 2013, 2013, 242149. Published online Jul 17, 2013. doi: 10.1155/2013/242149.

Ali, MAM. The Hypochromic Anemias. *Can Fam Physician.*, 1976, 22, 42–46.

Attivissimo, LA; Lichtman, SM; Klein, I. Acquired von Willebrand's syndrome causing a hemorrhagic diathesis in a patient with hypothyroidism. *Thyroid.*, 1995 Oct, 5(5), 399-401.

Bakkum-Gamez, JK; Laughlin, S; Jensen, J; Akogyeram, C; Pruthi, S. Challenges in the Gynecologic Care of Premenopausal Women With Breast Cancer Mayo Clin Proc., 2011, 86(3), 229–240.

Ballard, KD; Seaman, HE; de Vries, CS; Wright, JT. Can symptomatology help in the diagnosis of endometriosis? Findings from a national case-control study--Part 1. *BJOG.*, 2008 Oct, 115(11), 1382-91.

Barlow, DH; Lumsden, MA; Fauser, BC; Terrill, P; Bestel, E. Individualized vaginal bleeding experience of women with uterine fibroids in the PEARL I randomized controlled trial comparing the effects of ulipristal acetate or placebo. *Hum Reprod.*, 2014, 29(3), 480-9.

Battersby, S; Critchley, HO; de Brum-Fernandes, AJ; Jabbour, HN. Temporal expression and signalling of prostacyclin receptor in the human endometrium across the menstrual cycle. *Reproduction.*, 2004 Jan, 127(1), 79-86.

Bergeron, C; Amant, F; Ferenczy, A. Pathology and physiopathology of adenomyosis. *Best Pract Res Clin Obstet Gynaecol.*, 2006 Aug, 20(4), 511-21.

Byams, VR; Kouides, PA; Kulkarni, R; Baker, JR; Brown, DL; Gill, JC; Grant, AM; James, AH; Konkle, BA; Maahs, J; Dumas, MM; McAlister, S; Nance, D; Nugent, D; Philipp, CS; Soucie, JM; Stang, E. Haemophilia Treatment Centres Network Investigators. Surveillance of female patients with inherited bleeding disorders in United States Haemophilia Treatment Centres. *Haemophilia.*, 2011 Jul, 17 Suppl 1, 6-13.

Carey, ET; El-Nashar, SA; Hopkins, MR; Creedon, DJ; Cliby, WA, Famuyide, AO. Pathologic characteristics of hysterectomy specimens in women undergoing hysterectomy after global endometrial ablation. *J Minim Invasive Gynecol.*, 2011, 18(1), 96-9.

Caserta, D; Ralli, E; Matteucci, E; Bordi, G; Mallozzi, M; Moscarini, M. Combined oral contraceptives: health benefits beyond contraception. *Panminerva Med.*, 2014, 56(3), 233-44.

Chimbira, TH; Anderson, ABM; Turnbull, AC. Relation between measured menstrual blood loss and patient's subjective assessment of loss, duration of bleeding, number of sanitary towels used, uterine weight and endometrial surface area. *Br J Obstet Gynaecol.*, 1980, 87, 603–9.

Clark, TJ. Outpatient hysteroscopy and ultrasonography in the management of endometrial disease. *Curr Opin Obstet Gynecol.*, 2004, 16(4), 305-11.

Critchley, HO; Warner, P; Lee, AJ; Brechin, S; Guise, J; Graham, B. Evaluation of abnormal uterine bleeding: comparison of three outpatient procedures within cohorts defined by age and menopausal status. *Health Technol Assess.*, 2004, 8(34), iii-iv, 1-139.

Davidson, KG; Dubinsky, TJ. Ultrasonographic evaluation of the endometrium in postmenopausal vaginal bleeding. *Radiol Clin North Am.*, 2003 Jul, 41(4), 769-80.

Dean-Jones, L. Menstrual Bleeding According to the Hippocrates and Aristotle. Transactions of the American Philological Association, 1989.

Della, Badia, C; Karini, H. Endometrial stromal sarcoma diagnosed after uterine morcellation in laparoscopic supracervical hysterectomy. *J Minim Invasive Gynecol.*, 2010, 17(6), 791-3.

Dilley, A; Drews, C; Miller, C; Lally, C; Austin, H; Ramaswamy, D; Lurye, D; Evatt, B. von Willebrand disease and other inherited bleeding disorders in women with diagnosed menorrhagia. *Obstet Gynecol.*, 2001, 97(4), 630-6.

Donnez, J; Tatarchuk, TF; Bouchard, P; Puscasiu, L; Zakharenko, NF; Ivanova, T; Ugocsai, G; Mara, M; Jilla, MP; Bestel, E; Terrill, P; Osterloh, I, Loumaye, E; PEARL, I, Study, Group. Ulipristal acetate versus placebo for fibroid treatment before surgery. *N Engl J Med.*, 2012, 366(5), 409-20.

Duckitt, K; Collins, S. Menorrhagia. Clin Evid (Online., 2012 Jan 18, 2012. pii: 0805.

Dutton, W. Psychological Factors in 155 Patients with Functional Uterine Bleeding. *Canad. Med. Ass. J.*, Feb. 20, 1965, vol. 92.

Erdemoglu, E; Güney, M; Karahan, N; Mungan, T. Expression of cyclooxygenase-2, matrix metalloproteinase-2 and matrix metalloproteinase-9 in premenopausal and postmenopausal endometrial polyps. *Maturitas.*, 2008 Mar 20, 59(3), 268-74

Federici, AB. Acquired von Willebrand syndrome associated with hypo*thyroid*ism: a mild bleeding disorder to be further investigated. *Semin Thromb Hemost.*, 2011, 37(1), 35-40.

Finn, CA. Menstruation: a nonadaptive consequence of uterine evolution. *Q Rev Biol*, 1998, 73(2), 163-73.

Finn, CA. Why do women menstruate? Historical and evolutionary review. 1. *Eur J Obstet Gynecol Reprod Biol.*, 1996, 70(1), 3-8.

Fleischer, AC; Kalemeris, GC; Machin, JE; Entman, SS; James, AE Jr. Sonographic depiction of normal and abnormal endometrium with histopathologic correlation. *J Ultrasound Med.*, 1986, 5(8), 445-52.

Fraser, IS. Menorrhagia due to myometrial hypertrophy: treatment with tamoxifen. *Obstet Gynecol.*, 1987 Sep, 70(3 Pt 2), 505-6.

Fraser, IS. Menorrhagia--a pragmatic approach to the understanding of causes and the need for investigations. *Br J Obstet Gynaecol.*, 1994, 101 Suppl 11, 3-7.

Fraser, IS; Critchley, HO; Munro, MG; Broder, M. Writing Group for this Menstrual Agreement Process Fertil Steril. A process designed to lead to international agreement on terminologies and definitions used to describe abnormalities of menstrual bleeding. 2007 Mar, 87(3), 466-76.

Ghosh, P; Gandhi, G; Kochhar, PK; Zutshi, V; Batra, S. Visual inspection of cervix with Lugol's iodine for early detection of premalignant & malignant lesions of cervix. *Indian J Med Res.*, Aug, 2012, 136(2), 265–271.

Guttinger, A; Critchley, H. Endometrial effects of intrauterine levonorgestrel. *Contraception*, 2007, 75, S93-8.

Hallberg, L; Hogdahl, A; Nilsson, L; Rybo, G. Menstrualblood loss: a population study. *Acta Obstet Gynecol Scand.*, 1966, 45, 320–51.

Hallberg, L; Nilsson, L. Determination of menstrual blood loss. *Scand J Clin Lab Invest*, 1964, 16, 244–8.

Harlow, SB; Campbell, OMR. Epidemiology of menstrual disorders in developing countries: a systematic review Article first published online: 15 DEC, 2003

Haynes, PJ; Hodgson, H; Anderson, ABM, Turnbull, AC. Measurement of menstrual blood loss in patients complaining of menorrhagia.

Huq, FY; Tvarkova, K; Arafa, A; Kadir, RA. Menstrual problems and contraception in women of reproductive age receiving oral anticoagulation. *Contraception.*, 2011, 84(2), 128-32.

Hurskainen, R. Managing drug resistant essential menorrhagia without hysterectomy. *Best Pract Res Clin Obstet Gynaecol.*, 2006, 20, 681-94. Review.

Ibrahim, R; Khan, A; Raza, S; Kafeel, M; Dabas, R; Haynes, E; Gandhi, A, Majumder, OL; Zaman, M. Triad of iron deficiency anemia, severe thrombocytopenia and menorrhagia-a case report and literature review. *Clin Med Insights Case Rep.*, 2012, 5, 23-7.

Inki, P. Long-term use of the levenorgestrel – releasing uterine system. *Best Pract Res Clin Obstet Gynaecol*, 2006 Oct, 20(5), 681-94.

Jabbour, HN; Sales, KJ; Smith, OP; Battersby, S; Boddy, SC. Prostaglandin receptors are mediators of vascular function in endometrial pathologies. *Mol Cell Endocrinol.*, 2006 Jun 27, 252(1-2), 191-200.

James, A; Matchar, DB; Myers, ER. Testing for von Willebrand disease in women with menorrhagia: a systematic review. *Obstet Gynecol.*, 2004 Aug, 104(2), 381-8.

Jensen, J; Nelson, A; Costales, A. Subject and clinician experience with the levonorgestrel-releasing intrauterine system. *Contraception.*, 2008, 77, 22-9.

Jones, A; Harris, AL. New Developments in angiogenesis:a major mechanism for tumour growth and target for therapy. *Cancer j Sci Am*, 1998, 4, 209-217.

Karlsson, TS; Marions, LB; Edlund, MG. Heavy menstrual bleeding significantly affects quality of life. *Acta Obstet Gynecol Scand.*, 2014 Jan, 93(1), 52-7.

Krassas, GE; Pontikides, N; Kaltsas, T; Papadopoulou, P; Paunkovic, J; Paunkovic, N; Duntas, LH. Disturbances of menstruation in hypothyroidism. m Clin Endocrinol (Oxf)., 1999, 50(5), 655-9.

Kuzmina, N; Palmblad, J; Mints, M. Predictive factors for the occurrence of idiopathic menorrhagia: evidence for a hereditary trait. *Mol Med Rep.*, 2011, 4(5), 935-9.

Lethaby, A; Irvine, G; Cameron, I. Cyclical progestogens for heavy menstrual bleeding. *Cochrane Database Syst Rev.*, 2008 Jan 23, (1), CD001016.

Li, X; Liu, X; Guo, SW. Clinical profiles of 710 premenopausal women with adenomyosis who underwent hysterectomy. *J Obstet Gynaecol Res.*, 2014 Feb, 40(2), 485-94.

Lockwood, CJ. Mechanisms of Normal and Abnormal Endometrial Bleeding. *Menopause.*, 2011, 18(4), 408–411.

Luukkainen, T. The levonorgestrel intrauterine system: therapeutic aspects. *Steroids.*, 2000, 65, 699-702.

Management of Menorrhagia. NICE guidelines, 2007

Marsh, EE; Brocks, ME; Ghant, MS; Recht, HS; Simon, M. Prevalence and knowledge of heavy menstrual bleeding among African American women. *Int J Gynaecol Obstet.*, 2014 Apr, 125(1), 56-9

Matchar, J; Myers, E. Testing for von Willebrand disease in women with menorrhagia: a systematic review. *Obstet Gynecol.*, 2004 Aug, 104(2), 381-8.

Mauer, AC; Khazanov, NA; Levenkova, N; Tian, S; Barbour, EM; Khalida, C; Tobin, JN; Coller, BS. Impact of sex, age, race, ethnicity and aspirin use on bleeding symptoms in healthy adults. *Thromb Haemost.*, 2011 Jan, 9(1), 100-8.

Mengerink, BB; van der Wurff, AA; Ter, Haar JF; van Rooij, IA, Pijnenborg, JM. Effect of undiagnosed deep adenomyosis after failed NovaSure endometrial ablation. *J Minim Invasive Gynecol.*, 2014, S1553-4650(14)01442-3.

Miller, JD; Lenhart, GM; Bonafede, MM; Basinski, CM; Lukes, AS, Troeger, KA. Cost effectiveness of endometrial ablation with the NovaSure® system versus other global ablation modalities and hysterectomy for treatment of abnormal uterine bleeding: US commercial and Medicaid payer perspectives. *Int J Women's Health.*, 2015, 7, 59-73.

Mints, M; Luksha, L; Kublickiene, K. Altered responsiveness of small uterine arteries in women with idiopathic menorrhagia. *Am J Obstet Gynecol.*, 2008, 199(6), 646.e1-5.

Moragianni, VA; Somkuti, SG. Profound hypothyroidism-induced acute menorrhagia resulting in life-threatening anemia. *Obstet Gynecol.*, 2007, 110(2 Pt 2), 515-7.

Okeke, TC; Ikeako, LC; Ezenyeaku, CC Endometriosis. *Niger J Med.*, 2011, 20(2), 191-9.

Osayande, AS; Mehulic, S. Diagnosis and initial management of dysmenorrhea. *Am Fam Physician.*, 2014, 89(5), 341-6.

Palacios, S. The management of iron deficiency in menometrorrhagia. *Gynecol Endocrinol.*, 2011, 27 Suppl 1, 1126-30.

Peake, LJ; Grover, SR; Monagle, PT; Kennedy, AD. Effect of warfarin on menstruation and menstrual management of the adolescent on warfarin. *J Paediatr Child Health.*, 2011, 47(12), 893-7.

Peipert, SJ; Soper, DE. Diagnostic Evaluation of Pelvic Inflammatory Disease. Infect Dis *Obstet Gynecol.*, 1994, 2(1), 38–48.

Perrot, N; Mergui, JL; Frey, I; Uzan, M. Menorrhagia after age 40. Contribution of ultrasonic examination. *Gynecol Obstet Fertil.*, 2002, 30(6), 523-31.

Revel, A; Shushan, A. Investigation of the infertile couple: hysteroscopy with endometrial biopsy is the gold standard investigation for abnormal uterine bleeding. *Hum Reprod.*, 2002 Aug, 17(8), 1947-9

Rybo, G. Menstrual blood loss in relation to parity and menstrual pattern. *Acta Obst Gynecol Scand.*, 1966, 45 Suppl 7, 25–45.

Rybo, G. Menstrual blood loss in relation to parity and menstrual pattern. *Acta Obst Gynecol Scand*, 1966, 45 Suppl 7, 25–45.

Sales, K; Jabbour, N. Cyclooxygenase enzymes and prostaglandins in pathology of the endometrium. *Reproduction.*, 2003, 126(5), 559-67.

Sambrook, AM; Bain, C; Parkin, DE. A randomised comparison of microwave endometrial ablation with transcervical resection of the endometrium: follow up at a minimum of 10 years. *BJOG.*, 2009 Jul, 116(8), 1033-7.

Sanders, YV; de Wee, EM; Meijer, K; Eikenboom, J; van der Bom, JG; Fijnvandraat, CJ; Laros-van Gorkom, BA; Cnossen, MH; Mauser-Bunschoten, EP; Leebeek, FW. [Von Willebrand disease in the Netherlands: the WiN study]. *Ned Tijdschr Geneeskd.*, 2014, 158, A6518.

Shapley, M; Jordan, K; Croft, PR. Increased vaginal bleeding and psychological distress: a longitudinal study of their relationship in the community. *BJOG.*, 2003 Jun, 110(6), 548-54.

Shapley, M; Jordan, K; Croft, PR. Why women consult with increased vaginal bleeding: a case-control study *Br J Gen Pract.*, 2002 Feb, 52(475), 108-13.

Shiota, M; Yasushi, Kotani, Y; Umemoto, M; Tobiume, T; Hoshiai, H. Indication for Laparoscopically Assisted Vaginal Hysterectomy. *JSLS*, 2011, 15(3), 343–345.

Slupik, RI. Managing adolescents with eating disorders. *Int J Fertil Womens Med.*, 1999 May-Jun, 44(3), 125-30.

Smith, OP; Jabbour, HN; Critchley, HO. Cyclooxygenase enzyme expression and E series prostaglandin receptor signalling are enhanced in heavy menstruation. *Hum Reprod.*, 2007 May, 22(5), 1450-6.

Smith, P; Bakos, O; Heimer, G; Ulmsten, U. Transvaginal ultrasound for identifying endometrial abnormality. *Acta Obstet Gynecol Scand.*, 1991, 70(7-8), 591-4.

Sonoda, Y; Zerbe, M; Smith, A; Lin, O; Barakat, RR; Hoskins, WJ. High incidence of positive peritoneal cytology in low-risk endometrial cancer treated by laparoscopically assisted vaginal hysterectomy. *Gynecol Oncol.*, 2001, 80(3), 378-82.

Suar, Çakı, K; Nazan, S; Emine, Z; Sema, Aylan, G. Screening Bleeding Disorders in Adolescents and Young Women with Menorrhagia. *Turk J Haematol.*, Jun, 2013, 30(2), 168–176.

Sule, G; Ergul, Aslan; Nezihe, Kizilkaya, Beji; Meltem, Mecdi. The Effects of Menorrhagia on Women's Quality of Life: A Case-Control Study. *ISRN Obstet Gynecol.*, 2013, 2013, 918179.

Sweet, MG; Schmidt-Dalton, TA; Weiss, PM; Madsen, KP. Evaluation and management of abnormal uterine bleeding in premenopausal women. *Am Fam Physician.*, 2012 Jan 1, 85(1), 35-43.

Sweet, MG; Schmidt-Dalton, TA; Weiss, PM; Madsen, KP. Evaluation and management of abnormal uterine bleeding in premenopausal women. *Am Fam Physician.*, 2012, 85(1), 35-43.

Tan, YH; Lethaby, A. Pre-operative endometrial thinning agents before endometrial destruction for heavy menstrual bleeding. *Cochrane Database Syst Rev.*, 2013, 15, 11.

Tanaka, E; Momoeda, M; Osuga, Y; Rossi, B; Nomoto, K, Hayakawa, M; Kokubo, K; Wang, ECY. Burden of menstrual symptoms in Japanese women – an analysis of medical care-seeking behavior from a survey-based study. *Int J Womens Health.*, 2014, 6, 11–23.

Taran, FA; Stewart, EA; Brucker, S. Adenomyosis: Epidemiology, Risk Factors, Clinical Phenotype and Surgical and Interventional Alternatives to Hysterectomy. *Geburtshilfe Frauenheilkd.*, 2013 Sep, 73(9), 924-931.

Tokyol, C; Aktepe, F; Dilek, FH; Sahin, O; Arioz, DT. Expression of cyclooxygenase-2 and matrix metalloproteinase-2 in adenomyosis and endometrial polyps and its correlation with angiogenesis. *Int J Gynecol Pathol.*, 2009 Mar, 28(2), 148-56.

Valentini, AL; Speca, S; Gui, B; Soglia, G; Miccò, M; Bonomo, L. Adenomyosis: from the sign to the diagnosis. Imaging, diagnostic pitfalls and differential diagnosis: a pictorial review. *Radiol Med.*, 2011 Dec, 116(8), 1267-87.

van Eijkeren, MA; Schotten, PC; Christiaens, GCML; Alsbach, GPJ; Haspels, AA. The alkaline haematin method for measuring menstrual blood loss: a modification and its clinical use in menorrhagia. *Eur J Obstet Gynecol Reprod Biol*, 1986, 22, 345–51.

Weeks, A. Menorrhagia and hypo*thyroid*ism Evidence supports association between hypothyroidism and menorrhagia, *BMJ.*, 2000, 320(7235), 649.

Wilansky, DL; Greisman, B. Early hypo*thyroid*ism in patients with menorrhagia. *Am J Obstet Gynecol.*, 1989, 160(3), 673-7.

In: Menorrhagia and Dysmenorrhea
Editor: Timothy M. Welch
ISBN: 978-1-63482-552-8

Chapter II

Management of Heavy Menstrual Bleeding

***Ovidiu Nicodin*[*,1], *Bogdan Panaite*[1], *Diana Badiu*[2], *Dan Navolan*[3], *Tony Hangan*[2] and *Marius Popa*[2]**

[1]Department of Gynecology, Central Military University Emergency Hospital Dr. Carol Davila, UMF Carol Davila, Bucharest, Romania,
[2]Medicine, Ovidius University of Constanta, Romania
[3]Department of Obstetrics-Gynecology and Neonatology, Victor Babes University of Medicine and Pharmacy Timisoara, City Emergency Clinical Hospital Timisoara, Romania

Abstract

The complaints of heavy menstrual bleeding (HMB) have a substantial impact on the gynecological services and in most of the cases, without any other disorders. Some treatment considerably improves the quality of life, being important to decide the assessment of the patients by providing the best treatment options. This guideline provides instructions on how to examine and treat women with menorrhagia. Despite this, symptoms can be extremely distressing and different treatments are currently available. The choice of treatment depends on symptoms as

[*] E-mail: ovnicodin@yahoo.com.

well as the known potential side effects and risks of medication. The present review outlines a diagnostic approach and concentrated on different medical therapies like combined oral contraceptive pills, oral progesterone and levonorgestrel-releasing intrauterine system in contrast with surgical management, like endometrial ablation, uterine artery embolization or hysterectomy. With an effective treatment management, it is possible to better achieve the diagnostics of HMB, although area for further research is highlighted.

Keywords: heavy menstrual bleeding, menorrhagia, treatment, medical therapies, hysterectomy

1. Introduction

Heavy menstrual bleeding (HMB) or menorrhagia represent nowadays a social and health condition. From clinically point of view is defined as blood loss more than 80 mL per menstrual cycle. To diagnose menorrhagia represent also a difficult issue, being first defined like a perception of menstrual blood loss (MBL). Interestingly, the correlation between MBL with physical life quality of women showed to be the main key in treatment option. More often, menstrual cycles can be irregular and periods can be heavy and/or painful, improving with age. Symptoms can often be managed and proper advice such as appropriate use of simple analgesics is encouraging [1]. However, many situations require the gynecologist intervention. Such situations would include cases where simple achievements are unhelpful or where the women has a different condition which impacts the treatment advice. Moreover, women with learning difficulties may find even normal menstruation difficult to manage due to pain, fear which may request intervention. The HMB has an overall prevalence of 3.0% in pre-menopausal women but higher risk nearly doubles to more than 5% in women over 50 years. Therefore, the aim for improving the treatment conditions of HMB should be focused on psychosocial aspects of the women [2].

2. Medical Treatment

In major of cases, the medical cause is easily identified and effective treatments could also be involved and further prescribed. The choice of treatment first depends on symptoms and then on advice regarding all the measures which should be taken into account. However, many women who have been referred to tertiary care have already tried all the simple and basic measures, and further intervention or treatment is often required [3]. The medical treatment usually involves combined oral contraceptive, progesterone and levonorgestrel system.

Combined Oral Contraceptive Pills (COCPs)

It is known that COCPs represent a basic treatment for irregular menses and menorrhagia, inhibiting the production of luteinizing hormone and follicle-stimulating hormone. They act on the hypothalamic-pituitary axis suppressing ovulation. The majority of COCPs are dosed at the same dose throughout the 21-day of treatment. COCPs are generally used in 21-day treatment cycles followed by a 7-day break, during which time endometrial breakdown. Such withdrawal bleeding is quite different from the bleeding that occurs after a natural ovulatory cycle. COCPs have also a number of side effects including mood changes, headaches, and breast tenderness [4, 5]. In this respect, one study found that COCPs could reduce until 43% the menstrual blood loss [6]. There are also cases in which COCP can be used continuously is symptoms are very distressing, affecting the women daily. This could be taken before starting any other treatment which involves surgery or chemotherapy. Usually Microgynon 30 is the most used in these cases. The women which present polycystic ovarian syndrome would require more anti-androgenic pills, such as desogestrel or gestodene. If taken correctly, COCP is the most convenient contraception form, reducing the risk of ovarian [7], endometrial [8] and colorectal cancer [9].

Oral Progesterone

In menstrual problems, oral progesterone is used which can be taken continuously in order to improve irregular or heavy periods. The involved mechanisms by which oral progestogen reduce blood loss are still not well understood [10], as well as the efficacy used on follicular or luteal phase [11]. Sometimes there are situations which require delaying the menstrual period, like for example in the cases of surgical or chemotherapy, or different examinations.

Progesterone is produced during the luteal phase being responsible for transformation of the endometrium. Bleeding usually occurs when endogenous levels of progesterone fall and ovulation do not occur. Many oral progesterone available vary in the potency and adverse effect and the process by which MBL is reduced is still under debate [12]. One study showed that Rnorethisterone had no effect on MBL [13]. Another study showed that norethisterone was not as effective as the nonsteroidal anti-inflammatory drugs (NSAIDs). When compared with danazol, the latter was more effective in MBL reduction. A comparison with tranexamic acid revealed that norethisterone was not superior, as it failed to produce a better reduction in MBL. Oral progesterone in contrast with a progesterone intrauterine system (IUS) showed a positive change in MBL [14].

Levonorgestrel Intrauterine System (LNG-IUS)

The levonorgestrel intra-uterine system (LNG-IUS or Mirena) is a T-shaped plastic frame and the most effective contraceptive which usually releases 20 μg levonorgestrel into the uterine cavity each day. LNG-IUS could prevent endometrial proliferation and can inhibit ovulation in approximately 25% of the cases [15]. It also can be used when first-line treatments have failed [16, 17]. One study sustains the fact that LNG-IUS could reduce blood loss until 70-90% [18]. Sometimes could cause heavy bleeding or amenorrhea [19] and can be used in endometriosis management [20]. The effects of the LNG-IUS are mostly locally, preventing endometrial proliferation. At women who have normal uteri, the LNG-IUS is not required, having in the view that uterine cavities are containing fibroids which could retain the device [21]. Interestingly, amenorrhea was detected in 30% of the women who used LNG-IUS [22, 23].

3. Surgical Management

The surgical treatment is applied usually when medical treatment was failed or in the cases that can't be applied. The line between medical and surgical treatments depends both on women's age and the way HMB is affecting the life of a women [24]. One study compared the long-term benefits of medical in contrast with surgical management and showed that surgical management of HMB has a slight advantage over medical treatment, which showed to diminish in time. Although surgery has an advantage over medical treatment, the reversible nature of medical treatment compared with surgery must be taken into account [25]. The surgical treatment usually involves endometrial ablation, uterine artery embolization and hysterectomy.

Endometrial Ablation

One decade ago, if medical treatment was failed in repairing HMB, a hysterectomy was the only option. Over the time, many surgical options have been enterprise. Usually, endometrial ablation removes the endometrum together with superficial myometrium. First time, the endometrial ablation was used in resecting the tissue with an electrosurgical loop [26]. Then, other methods were used like thermal balloon endometrial ablation, bipolar radiofrequency including endometrial cryotherapy. Interestingly, these methods showed not to use direct uterine visualization when they are applied [27].

Uterine Artery Embolization (UAE)

Sometimes, the cause of HMB is the presence of fibroids. In these cases, the surgical option is uterine artery embolization (UAE). The UAE is used by an radiologist using small polyvinyl particles into the uterine arteries with the help of a catheter. The eventual loss of the blood supply to the fibroids allows us to efficiently treat HMB. Most often, UAE represent a safety procedure which requires shorter hospitalization. Into one study, based on the re-interventions, the myomectomy and other surgical techniques were applied instead of UAE [28]. Another study showed that after 1 year a greater reduction in menorrhagia was seen in the UAE surgical technique in contrast with the myomectomy technique [29].

Hysterectomy

In the case of menorrhagia, hysterectomy represents a final cure. By hysterectomy, the uterus is removed and before new other treatments were approved, this was the only viable treatment. In time, the hysterectomy seen to produce most of the morbidities, and it was taken the decision to reduce the number of this surgical technique. Other techniques were then approach like LNG-IUS, and endometrial ablation including UAE [30]. Therefore, based on the new applied techniques in the management of HMB, the number of hysterectomies has been decreased. Furthermore, advances in endoscopic technologies such as laser have enabled most hysterectomies to be performed with minimally invasive techniques. More conservative, effective, medical interventions should be better developed for alternatives to hysterectomy [31].

4. Duration of Therapy Preferences

Before starting any treatment, all the patients should be informed about the different options. Moreover, clinicians should inform about the length of the treatment chosen by any patient. LNG-IUD is most proper for the patients who do not want a daily oral regimen and are not planning to conceive in the next year. COCPs are available for the patients who prefer a daily regimen. Cyclin progestin may be offered to patients who prefer a monthly two-week treatment and NSAIDs may be suitable for the patients who desire a very short treatment [32].

Conclusion

Many women are affected by menorrhagia. Therefore, treatment options to control and manage the HMB are also available starting from medical to surgical techniques. Clinicians sustain the fact that menorrhagia is often incorrectly treated and further clinical trials are needed. With the development of new medical and surgical treatment options, further minimally invasive alternatives should become available.

References

[1] Parker M.; Sneddon A.; Arbon P. (2010). The menstrual disorder of teenagers (MDOT) study: determining typical menstrual patterns and menstrual disturbance in a large populationbased study of Australian teenagers. *BJOG, 117*, 185–192.

[2] Abbott J. (2002). Immediate endometrial resection for menorrhagia was more effective in the long term than initial medical management [Commentary]. Evidence-based. *Obstet.Gynecol., 4*, 126-7.

[3] Warner P.E.; Critchley H.O.; Lumsden M.A.; Campbell-Brown M.; Douglas A.; Murray G.D. (2004). Menorrhagia I: measured blood loss, clinical features, and outcome in women with heavy periods: a survey with follow-up data. *Am.J.Obstet.Gynecol., 190*, 1216-23.

[4] Fraser I.S.; McCarron G. (1991). Randomized trial of 2 hormonal and 2 prostaglandin-inhibiting agents in women with a complaint of menorrhagia. *Aust.N.Z.J.Obstet.Gynaecol., 31*, 66-70.

[5] Farquhar C.; Brown J. (2009). Oral contraceptive pill for heavy menstrual bleeding. *Cochrane Database Syst.Rev., 4*, CD000154.

[6] Miller L.; Hughes J.P. (2003). Continuous combination oral contraceptive pills to eliminate withdrawal bleeding: a randomized trial. *Obstet.Gynecol., 101*, 653-61.

[7] Bourdrez P.; Bongers M.Y.; Mol B.W. (2004). Treatment of dysfunctional uterine bleeding: patient preferences for endometrial ablation, a levonorgestrel-releasing intrauterine device, or hysterectomy. *Fertil.Steril., 82*, 160-6.

[8] Lethaby A.; Shepperd S.; Cooke I.; Farquhar C. (1999). Endometrial resection and ablation versus hysterectomy for heavy menstrual bleeding. *Cochrane Database Syst.Rev., 2*, CD000329.

[9] Fernandez E.; La Vecchia C.; Balducci A.; Chatenoud L.; Franceschi S.; Negri E. (2001). Oral contraceptives and colorectal cancer risk: a meta-analysis. *Br.J.Cancer, 84*, 722-7.

[10] Hallberg L.; Hogdahl A.M.; Nilsson L.; Rybo G. (1996). Menstrual blood loss- population study. Variation at different ages and attempts to define normality. *Acta Obstet.Gynecol.Scand., 45*, 320-51.

[11] Irvine GA.; Campbell-Brown M.B.; Lumsden M.A.; Heikkilä A.; Walker J.J.; Cameron I.T. (1998). Randomised comparative trial of the levon.orgestrel intrauterine system and norethisterone for treatment of idiopathic menorrhagia. *B.J.O.G., 105*, 592–598.

[12] Shapley M.; Jordan K.; Croft PR. (2003). Increased vaginal bleeding and psychological distress: a longitudinal study of their relationship in the community. *B.J.O.G., 110*, 548-54.

[13] Coulter A.; Kelland J.; Peto V.; Rees MC. (1995). Treating menorrhagia in primary care: an overview of drug trials and a survey of prescribing practice. *Int.J.Technol Assess Health Care, 11*, 456-71.

[14] Lethaby A.; Augood C.; Duckitt K. (1998). Nonsteroidal anti-inflammatory drugs for heavy menstrual bleeding. *Cochrane Database Syst.Rev., 3*, CD000400.

[15] Nilsson C.G.; Lähteenmäki P.L.A.; Luukkainen T. (1984). Ovarian function in amenorrheic and menstruating users of a levonorgestrel-releasing intrauterine device. *Fertil.Steril., 41*, 52-5.

[16] Thompson B.L.; Ponce de Leon R.; Kieke B.; Velebil P.; Wingo P.A. (1997). Trends in hospitalizations for abnormal uterine bleeding in the United States: 1980–1992. *J.Women's Health., 6,* 73-81.

[17] Liu Z.; Doan Q.V.; Blumenthal P.; Dubois R.W. (2007). A systematic review evaluating health-related quality of life, work impairment, and healthcare costs and utilization in abnormal uterine bleeding. *Value Health., 10*, 183-94.

[18] Stewart A.; Cummins C.; Gold L. et al., (2001). The effectiveness of the levonorgestrel-releasing intrauterine system in menorrhagia: a systematic review. *B.J.O.G., 108*, 74-86.

[19] Fraser I.S.; Critchley H.O.; Munro H.G.; Broder M. (2007). A process designed to lead to international agreement on terminologies and definitions to be used to describe abnormalities of menstrual bleeding. *Fertil.Steril., 87*, 466-76.

[20] Vercellini P.; Frontino G.; De Giorgi O.; Aimi G.; Zaina B.; Crosignani P.G. (2003). Comparison of a levonorgestrel-releasing intrauterine device versus expectant management after conservative surgery for symptomatic endometriosis: a pilot study. *Fertil.Steril., 80*, 305-9.

[21] Ballard K.D.; Seaman H.E.; de Vries C.S.; Wright JT. (2008). Can symptomatology help in the diagnosis of endometriosis? Findings from a national case-control study- Part 1. *B.J.O.G., 115*, 1382-91.

[22] Lethaby A.E.; Cooke I.; Rees M. (2000). Progesterone/progestogen releasing intrauterine systems for heavy menstrual bleeding. *Cochrane Database Syst.Rev., 2*, CD002126.

[23] Shaaban M.M.; Zakherah M.S.; El-Nashar S.A. et al., (2011). Levonorgestrel-releasing intrauterine system compared to low dose combined oral contraceptive pills for idiopathic menorrhagia: a randomized clinical trial. *Contraception, 83*, 48-54.

[24] Abbott J.A.; Garry R. (2002). The surgical management of menorrhagia. *Hum.Reprod.Update*, 8, 68-78.

[25] Marjoribanks J.; Lethaby A.; Farquhar C. (2006). Surgery versus medical therapy for heavy menstrual bleeding. *Cochrane Database Syst.Rev., 2*, CD003855.

[26] Lethaby A.; Hickey M.; Garry R. (2005). Endometrial destruction techniques for heavy menstrual bleeding. *Cochrane Database Syst.Rev., 4*, CD001501.

[27] Dilley A.; Drews C.; Miller C. et al., (2001). von Willebrand disease and other inherited bleeding disorders in women with diagnosed menorrhagia. *Obstet.Gynecol., 97*, 630-6.

[28] Gupta J.K.; Sinha A.S.; Lumsden M.A.; Hickey M. (2006). Uterine artery embolisation for symptomatic uterine fibroids. *Cochrane Database Syst.Rev., 1*, CD005073.

[29] Munro M.G.; Critchley H.O.; Broder M.S.; Fraser I.S. (2011). FIGO classification system (PALM-COEIN) for causes of abnormal uterine bleeding in nongravid women of reproductive age. *Int.J.Gynaecol.Obstet., 113*, 3-13.

[30] Learman L.A.; Summitt R.L.Jr.; Varner R.E.; Richter H.E.; Lin F.; Ireland C.C. et al., (2004). Hysterectomy versus expanded medical treatment for abnormal uterine bleeding: clinical outcomes in the medicine or surgery trial. *Obstet.Gynecol., 103*(5 pt 1), 824-33.

[31] Sowter M.C.; Lethaby A.; Singla A.A. (2002). Pre-operative endometrial thinning agents before endometrial destruction for heavy menstrual bleeding. *Cochrane Database Syst.Rev., 3*, CD001124.

[32] Philipp C.S.; Faiz A.; Dowling N.; Dilley A.; Michaels LA.; Ayers C. et al., (2005). Age and prevalence of bleeding disorders in women with menorrhagia. *Obstet.Gynecol., 105*, 61-6.

In: Menorrhagia and Dysmenorrhea
Editor: Timothy M. Welch
ISBN: 978-1-63482-552-8

Chapter III

The Role of Endometrial Inflammation in the Pathogenesis of Menorrhagia and the Clinical Use of NF-Kappa.b Natural Inhibitors with Hormone Therapy

***Hugo Maia Jr.*[1], *Clarice Haddad*[1], *Wilson SD dos Santos Junior*[2] *and Julio Casoy*[3]**

[1]Instituto da Mulher, Itaigara Memorial Day Hospital, Salvador, Bahia, Brazil
[2]Universidade do Estado da Bahia (UNEB), Department of Life Sciences, Salvador, Bahia, Brazil
[3]CEPARH, Salvador, Bahia, Brazil

Overview: Menstruation, Inflammation and the Role of Progesterone

Menstruation is an inflammatory process initiated by progesterone withdrawal, which elicits activation of the N-Kappa.b pathway. This triggers a complex inflammatory cascade involving the transcription of several genes coding for enzymes and inflammatory cytokines [1]. Among the essential enzymes involved in this pathway are the cyclooxygenase enzymes, responsible for the synthesis of several prostaglandins, which play a pivotal role in the mechanism of menstrual bleeding and pain.

However, other inflammatory mediators also play a pivotal role in the process of endometrial breakdown, remodeling and bleeding, which are important steps in the menstruation process. Angiogenic factors such as VEGF whose synthesis depends on the activation of the NF-kappa.b pathway also play an important role in the regulation of the amount of menstrual bleeding and pain [1, 2]. The intensity of these events is likewise affected by the quantity of proinflammatory prostaglandins and cytokines that are produced in the endometrium following progesterone withdrawal. This endometrial synthesis of prostaglandins will not only ultimately regulate the amount of bleeding and pain during menstruation but in susceptible patients will also activate the transcription of the aromatase gene in this tissue, thus stimulating local estrogen production [3-5]. This will further exacerbate cyclooxygenase activity, which in turn will generate more prostaglandins, thus establishing a vicious cycle of enhanced inflammation and enhanced estrogen production [1].

These disturbances in the endometrial metabolism of estrogens may be the underlying cause of functional menorrhagia and primary dysmenorrhea. There is also evidence that these functional changes may predate the development of pathologies such as adenomyosis, myomas, endometrial polyps and endometriosis, which would be the later consequences of this chronic exposure of the endometrium to locally synthesized estradiol and to the increased quantities of inflammatory mediators produced in this tissue in response to these changes in estrogen metabolism [1]. In all these pathologies, an increase in NF-kappa.b activation in the endometrium is consistently observed, showing a positive correlation with the amount of aromatase expression detected in this tissue [1, 6-8]

The importance of this estrogen-dependent inflammatory mechanism in the pathogenesis of menorrhagia and dysmenorrhea can be perceived when progestins are used to treat these conditions. When given continuously, these hormones effectively inhibit not only NF-Kappa.b activation in the endometrium but also aromatase, Cox-2 and VEGF expression in this tissue [1, 9-11]. This inhibitory effect is greatly augmented if natural NF-Kappa.b and aromatase inhibitors are administered concomitantly with hormone therapy, thus resulting in greater reductions in the quantity of uterine bleeding and dysmenorrhea when these combined treatments are used [1]. Recent studies have shown that in patients with menorrhagia who were using oral contraceptives in continuous regimens to treat this condition, the presence of persistent bleeding during treatment was associated with unabated aromatase expression in the endometrium [12]. In patients who developed amenorrhea, on the other hand, the expression of this enzyme became negative during treatment. These results show that aromatase expression is associated with the persistence of menstrual bleeding, thus suggesting that locally produced estrogens and heightened inflammation play a pivotal role in the pathogenesis of menorrhagia and dysmenorrhea. The use of plant-derived antioxidants such as pycnogenol is effective for the treatment of the pain and bleeding that persist during the use of oral contraceptives in patients with endometriosis [13]. As these flavonoids are also inhibitors of aromatase activity, their efficacy may also be a consequence of the blockade of this enzyme, thereby decreasing local estrogen production and heightened inflammation [1].

The Role of Inflammation and Local Estrogen Production in the Etiology of Menorrhagia

Aromatase expression can be detected in the endometrium of patients with menorrhagia even in the absence of any uterine pathology, thus suggesting that these functional changes may predate the development of pathology [12]. In this study, the percentage of endometria that were positive for aromatase expression did not differ significantly between patients with idiopathic menorrhagia and those with adenomyosis, thus suggesting that the mechanisms involved in the pathogenesis of excessive uterine bleeding may be the same, irrespective of the presence of pathology. One study conducted in primates showed that estradiol administered locally into the uterine cavity was able to provoke the development of several uterine pathologies including adenomyosis [14]. This suggests that there is probably a sequence of events occurring between the chronic exposure of the endometrium to locally synthesized estradiol and the future development of estrogen-dependent pathologies whose main presenting clinical symptom is menorrhagia. The local administration of estrogens may imitate the conditions found in the endometria of patients in whom aromatase expression is abnormally expressed [1]. This local endometrial production will create a hyperestrogenic milieu in the uterus that will antagonize the effect on progesterone in this tissue. This progesterone resistance will exacerbate inflammation in the endometrium by up-regulating Cox-2 and VEGF activity [1, 15]. This augmented prostaglandin production will initially exacerbate menstrual bleeding and dysmenorrhea and then go on to promote the development of adenomyosis and other estrogen-dependent pathologies that cause menorrhagia [1]. In patients with this menstrual symptom, the intensity of Cox-2 expression in the endometrium did not differ significantly between those with a normal uterus and those with adenomyosis [12]. This is in agreement with the hypothesis that the mechanisms responsible for excessive menstrual bleeding are similar in both normal and pathology-bearing uteri, since in both conditions there is an increased production of estrogens in the endometrium which causes an exacerbation of inflammation in this tissue [1]. In this respect, idiopathic menorrhagia and primary dysmenorrhea could be the first manifestations of increased endometrial inflammation triggered by an aberrant local estrogen production up-regulating the cyclooxygenase enzyme responsible for the synthesis of proinflammatory prostaglandins [1].

It is tempting to speculate that menorrhagia occurring either in the presence of normal uteri or in association with pathology may represent different stages of the same functional changes that occur in the endometrium. Initially they would cause only an increase in menstrual bleeding and pain but if left untreated they would provoke the development of various estrogen-dependent pathologies [1]. Unfortunately, it is difficult to assess from clinical observations whether aromatase expression predates the development of adenomyosis or other pathologies, since it not ethical to leave patients initially diagnosed with idiopathic menorrhagia untreated to see whether they will go on to develop uterine pathology. However, in patients with idiopathic menorrhagia treated initially with endometrial resection but who had to endure a second procedure because of a recurrence of the menorrhagia, the pathology report from the second procedure showed the presence of adenomyosis in uteri that were originally pathology-free [16]. This is in agreement with the idea that chronic exposure of the endometrium to locally produced estradiol will initially cause excessive menstrual bleeding by up-regulating Cox-2 expression, only later provoking the development of pathology. However, it is impossible to conclude from these uncontrolled observations whether the trauma associated with endometrial resection could have contributed to the development of adenomyosis by disrupting the endometrial myometrial architecture.

Aromatase expression in the endometrium increases not only with the severity of endometriosis but also when adenomyosis is present, since this pathology is commonly associated with the most advanced stages of the disease [17]. The augmented expression of aromatase in the endometrium of these patients is the result of an increase in the number of mRNA transcripts for this enzyme, thus suggesting that epigenetic changes leading to enhanced gene transcription may be the underlying mechanism that triggers the development of this pathology [1, 17].

In patients with a history of menorrhagia who were experiencing breakthrough bleeding during the use of oral contraceptives in continuous regimens, aromatase expression could still be detected in their endometrium, while in those who achieved amenorrhea during treatment the expression of this enzyme became negative [12]. The unabated aromatase expression in the endometrium of these patients was probably the consequence of a functional resistance to the action of the progestin present in the composition of these contraceptive pills which impeded the inhibition of both Cox-2 and NF-Kappa.b activity by these hormones [9]. The persistent aromatase expression in the endometrium maintains Cox-2 and NF-Kappa.b activity unabated and this may be the mechanism that triggers the occurrence of breakthrough bleeding and dysmenorrhea in these patients [1, 9, 12]. These findings are in agreement with the hypothesis that as long as aromatase expression remains positive amenorrhea is not achieved and the menstrual-related symptoms remain unresolved because inflammation continues unabated in the endometrium [1].

Several progestins commonly used in the treatment of menorrhagia and dysmenorrhea are capable of slowing down aromatase expression in endometrial cells by acting at gene transcription level [11, 18, 19]. However, it remains to be established whether this is a direct inhibitory effect of progestin on the DNA regulatory regions or the indirect consequence of halting inflammation in the tissue [1]. Local estrogen production in the endometrium may be the mechanism responsible for the occurrence of menorrhagia and dysmenorrhea, irrespective of the presence of pathology in the uterus, since the ensuing hyperestrogenism can lead to an increased inflammatory milieu [1]. From a biological point of view, this is a plausible possibility, as the increased local estrogen production in the endometrium will up-regulate Cox-2 expression, thus stimulating a great production of proinflammatory prostaglandins, which in turn will exacerbate menstrual bleeding and pain [1, 20]. These proinflammatory prostaglandins may subsequently stimulate the transcription of the aromatase gene in some susceptible women, thus increasing local estrogen production, which, in turn, will incite further Cox-2 activity [1]. The resulting continuation of aromatase and Cox-2 expression in the endometrium may ultimately be responsible for the development of a progesterone resistance in this tissue [1]. These findings also explain why the use of oral contraceptives in continuous regimens in conjunction with plant-derived aromatase inhibitors such as resveratrol is associated with a lesser incidence of breakthrough bleeding and pain in patients with endometriosis compared to the use of oral contraceptives alone [21].

In conclusion, it has been suggested that local estrogen production in the endometrium may play a pivotal role in increasing menstrual flow, thus constituting the underlying mechanism responsible for the development of idiopathic menorrhagia. The time sequence of enhanced aromatase expression in the endometrium occurring prior to the subsequent development of any pathology may explain the long delay between the onset of menstrual symptoms and the clinical diagnosis of these estrogen-dependent pathologies. The increase in local estrogen production is positively associated with the exacerbation of menstrual symptoms such as bleeding and pain and they may occur either prior to or in association with a uterine pathology.

The Association of Natural NF-Kappa.b Inhibitors with Oral Contraceptives in the Treatment of Menorrhagia

The aromatase gene is activated in the endometrium by proinflammatory prostaglandin E2, which is generated in tissues as a result of Cox-2 activity. Since this is an NF-Kappa.b inducible gene, aromatase expression may depend on the inflammatory status of the tissues [22]. Adenomyosis and endometriosis are examples of estrogen-dependant inflammatory pathologies in which NF-Kappa.b is constitutively expressed in the endometrium [7, 8]. The constant activation of NF-Kappa.b in patients with adenomyosis and its binding to the DNA responsive elements enhances transcription of the cyclooxygenase gene, thus boosting aromatase gene expression in response to the increased exposure to inflammatory prostaglandins [1, 23]. The increase in cyclooxygenase gene expression is associated with menorrhagia. Progestins such as gestodene or dienogest can effectively block NF-Kappa.b DNA binding activity by preventing its translocation to cell nucleus; therefore, they effectively treat menorrhagia and halt inflammation. This inhibits the initiation of the inflammatory cascade that will ultimately provoke transcription of the aromatase gene [1].

In pathology free uteri, aromatase expression is associated with the presence of menorrhagia and dysmenorrhea. The presence of breakthrough bleeding during the continuous use of oral contraceptives is the consequence of unabated NF-Kappa.b activity, which, in turn, will augment the transcription of several genes directly or indirectly related to the inflammatory cascade, such as the cyclooxygenase gene [19]. The presence of high inflammatory status in the endometrium will maintain the transcription of the aromatase gene active [1]. This will increase estrogen production in the endometrium, which will further enhance cyclooxygenase activity, thus stimulating a vicious cycle of increased inflammation and estrogen production that is pivotal in stimulating the over-production of angiogenic factors such as VEGF, ultimately leading to menorrhagia [1]. In fact, there is a positive correlation between the intensity of VEGF and Cox-2 production in the endometrium and the severity of menorrhagia and dysmenorrhea [1, 24, 25].

The complete suppression of aromatase expression following hormone treatment is therefore necessary to achieve amenorrhea and increase the pain-free intervals in patients with endometriosis and adenomyosis. Treatments that combine oral contraceptives with an association of natural NF-Kappa.b and aromatase inhibitors may prove more beneficial than their use alone, since this combination may increase the efficacy of treatment without increasing side effects by further decreasing inflammation in the endometrium [13, 21]. The combination of resveratrol and oral contraceptives effectively suppressed aromatase expression in the endometrium of patients with endometriosis while also increasing amenorrhea rates and dysmenorrhea-free intervals [21].

Other plant-derived NF-Kappa.b inhibitors such as pycnogenol, a mixture of flavonoids extracted from the bark of a maritime pine tree (pinus pinaster), are likewise effective for the treatment of dysmenorrhea when used either alone or in association with oral contraceptives [13]. The latter regimen proved to be more effective in inducing amenorrhea and decreasing pain in endometriosis patients compared to the use of contraceptives alone. Pycnogenol also potentiated the inhibitory effects of oral contraceptives on aromatase and VEGF expression in the endometrium of myomatous uteri. One plausible explanation is the blockade of NF-Kappa.b activity by pycnogenol, which would decrease inflammation further, thus leading to a greater reduction in aromatase activity in the endometrium. This would exert an additional inhibitory effect on aromatase expression, potentiating the inhibition of the aromatase gene transcription through the use of oral contraceptives [26-28]. Since aromatase expression in the endometrium may serve as a marker of the severity of endometriosis, the greater inhibition of this enzyme with the combination of continuous oral contraceptives and either resveratrol or pycnogenol would potentiate the efficacy of oral contraceptives in the treatment of endometriosis, adenomyosis and myomas.

The effects of the pinus pinaster extract could be further potentiated with the concomitant use of resveratrol to inhibit aromatase activity in endometriosis patients using oral contraceptives, since these two products act in different steps. Resveratrol is able to inhibit aromatase at both enzyme and mRNA levels, while the flavonoids present in the pinus pinaster extract act indirectly by suppressing inflammation through the reduction of NF-Kappa.b translation of inflammatory genes after its binding to DNA [26, 27]. Furthermore, it has recently been reported that resveratrol is likewise able to diminish inflammation by inhibiting nuclear translocation of NF-kappa.b p65 by preventing its translocation to cell nuclei [28]. This suggests that combining resveratrol with pinus pinaster extract could result in a more effective inhibition of NF-Kappa.b activity by acting not only prior to its binding to DNA but also after this event. This would result in less inflammation and aromatase expression in the endometrium.

Our group recently studied the effect of the combination of resveratrol with pinus pinaster extract on aromatase expression in the endometrium of endometriosis patients undergoing treatment with oral contraceptives in continuous regimens (Maia Jr. H, unpublished results). These patients had pain and menorrhagia. The study population consisted of 175 patients referred to our center for diagnostic hysteroscopy with endometrial biopsy. The patients were divided into five groups according to the treatment they were receiving at the time of hospital admission: Group A: 48 patients with a history of pelvic pain and/or infertility and no hormonal treatment; Group B: 36 patients using oral contraceptives in extended regimens; Group C: 46 endometriosis patients who had been using oral contraceptives together with 100 mg of a pinus pinaster extract and 30 mg of resveratrol daily; Group D: 15 patients using only the pinus pinaster extract with resveratrol; and Group E: 30 patients using oral contraceptives with resveratrol. Aromatase expression was determined in the endometrium by immunohistochemistry. Our results showed that aromatase activity was detected in the stroma of patients in the untreated control group (Group A) with endometriosis/adenomyosis. When the proliferative and secretory phases of the menstrual cycle were compared, no statistically significant difference was found in the incidence of aromatase-positive endometria (80% versus 78%, respectively); therefore, both phases of the cycles were evaluated together.

The use of oral contraceptives in extended regimens prior to hospital admission was associated with a significant reduction in the percentage of endometrial stroma showing positive aromatase expression. In this group, the mean number of aromatase-positive cases decreased significantly to 50% ($p=0.005$) after a mean duration of pill use of two months. In Group C, the combination of oral contraceptives in extended regimens with pinus pinaster extract + resveratrol caused a further reduction in the positivity for aromatase expression in the endometrium. In this group, the mean percentage of positive staining in the stroma was only 6%, which was significantly lower than that of Groups A and B ($p<0.0001$). In Group D, which consisted of patients using pinus pinaster extract + resveratrol but who did not use oral contraceptives, the mean percentage of positive aromatase expression was significantly lower than in Group A (the control group) ($p=0.01$) but not different from those using oral contraceptives alone (Group B). However, it was significantly higher than in Group C ($p=0.0002$). In patients using oral contraceptives with resveratrol (Group E), the percentage of positive aromatase expression was still significantly higher than in Group C but lower than in Group B, although this difference failed to reach statistical significance ($p=0.07$). These results are summarized in Table 1.

Table 1. Percentage of cases in which the endometrium of patients with endometriosis was found to be positive for aromatase expression

Group A	Untreated patients	34/48	79%
Group B	Users of oral contraceptives alone	18/36	50%
Group C	Oral contraceptives + pinus pinaster + resveratrol	3/46	6%
Group D	Pinus pinaster + resveratrol	7/15	47%
Group E	Oral contraceptives + resveratrol	10/30	33%

Group A x Group B	$p = 0.005$
Group A x Group C	$p<0.0001$
Group A x Group D	$p = 0.01$
Group B x Group C	$p<0.000001$
Group B x Group D	Not significant
Group C x Group D	$p = 0.000$

The concomitant use of pinus pinaster extract + resveratrol with oral contraceptives (Group C) was associated with a decrease in the percentage of patients reporting breakthrough bleeding and pain. These symptoms were reported by 15/36 patients in Group B (41%) and by only 7/46 in Group C (15%) (p=0.04).

This decrease in the incidence of symptoms in Group C was associated with the more effective inhibition of aromatase expression in the eutopic endometrium. When patients in Groups B and C were analyzed together, the percentage of positive aromatase expression was found to be 68% in the endometria of symptomatic patients compared to only 4% in the asymptomatic women. This difference was statistically significant (p=0.00006).

These results showed that treatments that combine oral contraceptives with this association of natural NF-Kappa.b and aromatase inhibitors may prove more beneficial than their use alone, since they may increase the efficacy of treatment without increasing side effects.

The combination of resveratrol and oral contraceptives effectively suppressed aromatase expression in the endometrium of endometriosis patients; however, adding pinus pinaster extract to this combination further potentiated the inhibitory effects of this treatment on the expression of this enzyme in the endometrium. One plausible explanation is the blockade of NF-Kappa.b activity by the pinus pinaster extract, which will further decrease inflammation, thus leading to a greater reduction in aromatase activity in the endometrium.

This will exert an additional inhibitory effect on aromatase expression, potentiating the direct inhibition of the aromatase gene transcription by resveratrol [29]. Since aromatase expression in the endometrium may serve as a marker of the severity of endometriosis, the findings reported here that the combination of resveratrol with pinus pinaster extract greatly potentiates the inhibitory effect of oral contraceptives suggest that combining hormone therapy with natural NF-kappa.b and aromatase inhibitors may be more beneficial for the treatment of menorrhagia and pain than the use of hormone therapy alone. However, well-designed double-blind clinical trials are necessary to prove or refute this hypothesis.

Perhaps in the future, the combination of hormone therapy with natural NF-kappa.b inhibitors may become the preferable treatment for menorrhagia and dysmenorrhea because of the greater inhibition of aromatase expression achieved. One of the genes whose transcription is activated following the binding of NF-kappa.b to DNA responsive elements is VEGF.

We had previously shown that oral contraceptives containing gestodene were effective in decreasing VEGF expression in patients with myomas [10]. Since both pycnogenol (pinus pinaster extract) and resveratrol inhibit NF-Kappa.b activation, it is possible that their use in combination with oral contraceptives may potentiate their inhibitory effect on VEGF. We have recently investigated this issue in patients with either endometriosis or myomas and with symptoms of menorrhagia and dysmenorrhea. In this group, the percentage of positive endometria for VEGF, evaluated using immunohistochemical methods, was 89%, with the endometrium testing negative in only 11% of cases (n=48). The staining reaction for VEGF was always detected in the endometrial stroma.

In patients using oral contraceptives (OCs) containing either gestodene or drospirenone in continuous regimens, the proportion of endometria testing negative for VEGF rose significantly from 10% in the untreated group to 35% (p=0.002). However in patients using OCs together with pinus pinaster extract (pycnogenol) + resveratrol (n=50), the percentage of negative endometria was 54% and this was significantly greater than in the other two groups. This suggests that pinus pinaster extract and resveratrol greatly potentiate the inhibitory effects of oral contraceptives on VEGF expression in the endometrium of patients with myomas and endometriosis.

We recently investigated the effect of resveratrol on uterine size and menorrhagia in patients with myomas who were using oral contraceptives in extended regimens. Because resveratrol decreases fibrosis by blocking TGF beta, it would be interesting to investigate whether it would affect myoma growth [30].

In this study, uterine size was determined by vaginal ultrasonography prior to and after six months of treatment. This study was conducted in 74 patients using oral contraceptives containing either drospirenone or gestodene, associated or not with resveratrol. The addition of 30 mg of oral resveratrol to the oral contraceptive regimen led to a reduction in uterine size in 70% of patients, while the administration of either OCs or resveratrol alone resulted in a smaller and nonsignificant increase in the number of patients showing a reduction in uterine size. The combination of resveratrol with oral contraceptives was also effective in treating menorrhagia associated with the presence of myomas. Following treatment, 90% of the patients became amenorrheic.

Hormonal Treatment of Menorrhagia and Dysmenorrhea with Vaginal Gestrinone Associated with Natural NF-Kappa.b Inhibitors

Adenomyosis is a common condition that frequently co-exists together with endometriosis, with a prevalence of 22% in patients with deep forms of this disease. In a recent study, it was found that in 217 patients with an ultrasonographic diagnosis of adenomyosis, 73 had ovarian endometriosis and 92 had deep infiltrating endometriosis [31], thus confirming the strong relationship that exists between adenomyosis and endometriosis. Myomas are also frequently associated with endometriosis [10]. Since these pathologies may cause abnormal uterine bleeding, the coexistence of menorrhagia and dysmenorrhea is a frequent clinical finding. Most of the hormonal treatments used for endometriosis are also effective in ameliorating menorrhagia. One of these hormones is gestrinone, which has been used for the treatment of endometriosis and myomas for more than three decades [32]. It is highly effective when administered by the oral route; however, its androgenic side effects precluded its wider acceptance.

Nonoral routes for the administration of gestrinone have been developed in Brazil, particularly in the form of subdermal implants [33]. Despite the lower incidence of androgenic side effects with the implants compared to the oral administration, subdermal implants have the disadvantage that their insertion and removal involve invasive procedures and doses cannot easily be adjusted by the patient once the implants are inserted [32, 33].

The development of simple, non-invasive and self-administered routes through which to deliver gestrinone may offer certain advantages over the use of implants for the treatment of menorrhagia and dysmenorrhea. One promising route is through the vaginal mucosa. Previous studies in the 1980s showed that the insertion of a 2.5 mg pill containing gestrinone into the vagina two or three times a week effectively managed pain in endometriosis patients and induced amenorrhea in almost 50% of patients, with fewer side effects when compared to either the oral or subdermal routes [33]. The vaginal mucosa appeared a promising alternative for the delivery of hormones for the treatment of uterine pathologies because of the first uterine pass effect, which concentrates a hormone in the pelvic organs and uterus before distributing it into the systemic circulation [34]. This is accomplished through an active transport mechanism which acts locally and is greatly helped by the close proximity of the vaginal vein and artery. This creates a concentration gradient in the pelvic organs that enables vaginally administered hormones to reach high tissue levels despite rather low systemic blood levels [32].

Recently, the development of better permeation excipients such as Pentravan™, which proved effective for the vaginal delivery of danazol to treat deep endometriosis-related pain, prompted us to investigate its use with gestrinone in association with a combination of natural polyphenols endowed with antioxidant and anti-inflammatory properties not only for pelvic pain but also for menorrhagia [35]. One such compound consists of a complex mixture of flavonoids extracted from the bark of a pine tree (pinus pinaster), which blocks NF-Kappa.b activity after its binding to DNA responsive elements. The effects of pinus pinaster extract may be further potentiated with the concomitant use of resveratrol to inhibit aromatase activity in endometriosis patients, since this enzyme plays a pivotal role in the progression of endometriosis [1, 13, 21].

We recently investigated the effect of a combination of vaginal gestrinone in Pentravan™ with oral pinus pinaster extract and resveratrol on pain scores and uterine bleeding in patients with endometriosis who also had concomitant adenomyosis or myomas. Pain was assessed using a visual analog pain scale at 1, 2 and 6 months after initiation of treatment. Prior to treatment, mean pain score was 9. Vaginal gestrinone in Pentravan™ significantly decreased the intensity of pain. This response was rapid and already observed in the first month of treatment. After the second month of treatment, almost 85% of the patients were pain free and the mean pain score decreased to 0.4. After the third month, all 35 patients enrolled in this clinical observation reported no pain at all. Gestrinone was not only effective for the treatment of dysmenorrhea, but the combination with the pinus pinaster extract and resveratrol, administered orally, induced amenorrhea after the second month of treatment in 90% of the patients. The cessation of menstrual bleeding was accompanied by a reduction in uterine volume not only in patients with endometriosis/adenomyosis but also in the case of myomas. In the latter, uterine volume decreased significantly (p=0.001) from 206 cm^3 to 138 cm^3 in the third month of treatment. In patients with adenomyosis/endometriosis, uterine volume reduced significantly from 146 cm^3 to 115 cm^3 (p=0.04). There was also a significant reduction in the volume of ovarian endometriotic cysts from 36 cm^3 to 18 cm^3 (p=0.004) after the third month of treatment.

Vaginal gestrinone did not significantly decrease baseline blood levels of either FSH or LH, although ovulation was suppressed in all patients using 5 mg of gestrinone vaginally three times a week. Blood levels of estradiol and total testosterone, on the other hand, decreased significantly. However, the decrease in total testosterone had no negative effect on libido, since there was a relative increase in free testosterone resulting from the considerable decrease in SHBG levels induced by the vaginal administration of gestrinone. SHBG levels decreased from 97 nmol/l to 12 nmol/L in the first three months of treatment. Other metabolic parameters were also affected by this treatment. A significant decrease in triglycerides, HDL cholesterol and glucose was observed. Total cholesterol levels and LDL, on the other hand, were not significantly affected. Because of the high rates of amenorrhea, there was a significant increase in hemoglobin levels, which was already apparent in the second month of treatment. The endometrium became thin and there was a considerable decrease in the density of the vascular network, giving the mucosa a pale, avascular appearance at hysteroscopy.

Table 2. Effect of vaginal gestrinone in Pentravan™ with oral pinus pinaster extract + resveratrol on metabolic and hormonal parameters

Variable	Baseline (mean ± SD)	After two months of treatment (mean ± SD)	Statistical significance
Glucose (mg/dl)	86 ± 9	76± 9	p=0.01
SHBG (nmol/1)	97 ± 60	12± 5	p = 0.001
Total cholesterol (mg/dl)	182 ± 35	174±	NS
HDL (mg/dl)	50 ± 10	28± 11	p<0.001
LDL (mg/dl)	118 ± 32	132 ± 62	NS
AST (U/l)	24 ±1 4	42± 54	NS
ALT (UI/l)	23± 7	38 ± 55	NS
LH (mIU/ml)	5 ± 3	4 ± 1	NS
FSH (mIU/ml)	9 ± 2	7 ± 4	NS
Estradiol (pg/ml)	113 ± 90	34 ± 22	p = 0.001
Total testosterone (ng/dl)	25 ± 7	18 ± 3	p = 0.001
Triglycerides (mg/dl)	106 ± 59	71 ± 27	p < 0.005
Hemoglobin (g/dl)	11.2 ± 1.5	12.5 ± 1	p = 0.007

SD: standard deviation; NS: not significant; SHBG: sex hormone binding globulin; HDL: high-density lipoprotein cholesterol; LDL: low-density lipoprotein cholesterol; ALT: alanine transaminase; AST: aspartate transaminase. FSH: Follicle Stimulating Hormone LH: Luteinizing Hormone.

Liver enzymes were not adversely affected by the treatment in the majority of the patients, with the exception of two cases (2/35) in which there was a rise in alanine transaminase (ALT) and in aspartate transaminase (AST) levels, which returned to normal after discontinuation of treatment. These results are summarized in Table 2.

Vaginal gestrinone in Pentravan™, when used in association with oral pinus pinaster and resveratrol, proved to be a very effective treatment for both pelvic pain and menorrhagia. The resolution of symptoms is accompanied by an actual decrease in both uterine volume and in the size of the myoma. Vaginal gestrinone decreased aromatase expression in the endometrium of patients with endometriosis after the first month of treatment. The blockade of aromatase activity may be one of the mechanisms involved in the pain and menorrhagia ameliorating effects of gestrinone. The antiestrogenic effects of gestrinone, which are mainly due to its androgenic effect and do not involve interaction with the estrogen receptors, may further inhibit endometrial proliferation and bleeding, thus contributing to the high rates of amenorrhea. This also explains the thin endometrium observed at transvaginal ultrasonography in patients using vaginal gestrinone despite the presence of ovarian follicles.

Vaginal gestrinone, administered in association with pinus pinaster extract and resveratrol, will halt inflammation, both in the endometrium and in the endometriotic lesions, and this will ultimately lead to the suppression of aromatase expression, the resolution of pain symptoms and the induction of amenorrhea. The inhibition of aromatase activity is a rather slow process and is only observed after the first months of treatment. It is probably a consequence of the reduction in endometrial inflammation rather than direct inhibition of gene transcription.

The incidence of androgenic side effects with the vaginal route appears to be lower than with the oral route and this may be due to the lower blood levels of gestrinone achieved with this route of administration [32, 33]. Although the reduction in SHBG levels may increase free testosterone levels, this may enhance the antiinflammatory effects of treatment, since testosterone has a negative effect on inflammation and a boosting effect on libido.

Testosterone is an inhibitor of NF-Kappa.b activation, and this explains the positive impact on the amelioration of pain and in the resolution of menorrhagia [36]. Contrary to other treatments for endometriosis that may adversely affect sexuality, this does not seem to occur with gestrinone. The therapeutic efficacy of gestrinone depends on its absorption through the vagina, which is greatly enhanced with the use of Pentravan™. This ultimately results in high concentrations of gestrinone in the pelvis, with lower systemic blood levels due to the uterine first pass effect [34]. The concomitant use of oral pinus pinaster extract with resveratrol will further decrease inflammation by blocking NF-Kappa.b activity and lowering the oxidative stress, not only locally in the lesions and endometrium but also systemically. This combined approach for the treatment of endometriosis and menorrhagia appears promising. The vaginal mucosa may be the best route for the delivery of active pharmacological agents for the treatment of menorrhagia because of the uterine first pass effect [34]. The use of Pentravan™ (Fagron, the Netherlands) to deliver these agents vaginally has proven effective ever since its first use with danazol for the treatment of endometriosis.

References

[1] Maia Jr. H, Haddad C, Coelho G, Casoy J. Role of inflammation and aromatase expression in the eutopic endometrium and its relationship with the development of endometriosis. *Womens Health.* 2012 Nov;8 (6): 647-58 (Review).

[2] Sugino N, Karube-Harada A, Taketani T, Sakata A, Nakamura Y. Withdrawal of ovarian steroids stimulates prostaglandin F2alpha production through nuclear factor-kappa.B activation via oxygen radicals in human endometrial stromal cells: potential relevance to menstruation. *J Reprod Dev.* 2004 Apr;50(2):215-25.

[3] Maia Jr. H, Casoy J, Valente Filho J. Is aromatase expression in the endometrium the cause of endometriosis and related infertility? *Gynecol Endocrinol.* 2009 Apr;25 (4): 253-7 (Review).

[4] Bulun SE, Noble LS, Takayama K, Michael MD, Agarwal V, Fisher C, Zhao Y, Hinshelwood MM, Ito Y, Simpson ER. Endocrine disorders associated with inappropriately high aromatase expression. *J Steroid Biochem Mol Biol.* 1997 Apr;61 (3-6): 133-9. Review. PubMed PMID: 9365182.

[5] Noble LS, Takayama K, Zeitoun KM, Putman JM, Johns DA, Hinshelwood MM, Agarwal VR, Zhao Y, Carr BR, Bulun SE. Prostaglandin E2 stimulates aromatase expression in endometriosis-derived stromal cells. *J Clin Endocrinol Metab.* 1997 Feb;82 (2): 600-6.

[6] González-Ramos R, Defrère S, Devoto L. Nuclear factor-kappaB: a main regulator of inflammation and cell survival in endometriosis pathophysiology. *Fertil Steril.* 2012;98(3):520-8.
[7] González-Ramos R, Rocco J, Rojas C, Sovino H, Poch A, Kohen P, Alvarado-Díaz C, Devoto L. Physiologic activation of nuclear factor kappa-B in the endometrium during the menstrual cycle is altered in endometriosis patients. *Fertil Steril.* 2012; 97 (3): 645-51.
[8] Donnez J. Involvement of the nuclear factor-κB pathway in the pathogenesis of endometriosis. *Fertil Steril.* 2010 Nov;94(6):1985-94.
[9] Maia H Jr, Casoy J, Correia T, Athayde C, Valente J, Coutinho EM. Activation of NF-kappaB and COX-2 expression is associated with breakthrough bleeding in patients using oral contraceptives in extended regimens. *Gynecol Endocrinol.* 2010; 26 (4): 265-9.
[10] Maia H Jr, Casoy J, Pimentel K, Correia T, Athayde C, Cruz T, Coutinho EM. Effect of oral contraceptives on vascular endothelial growth factor, Cox-2 and aromatase expression in the endometrium of uteri affected by myomas and associated pathologies. *Contraception* 2008; 78 (6): 479-85.
[11] Maia H Jr., Casoy J, Correia T, Freitas LA, Pimentel K, Athayde C. The effect of oral contraceptives on aromatase expression in the eutopic endometrium of patients with endometriosis. *Gynecol Endocrinol.* 2008; 24 (3): 123-8.
[12] Maia H Jr, Haddad C, Pinheiro N, Casoy J. The effect of oral contraceptives on aromatase and Cox-2 expression in the endometrium of patients with idiopathic menorrhagia or adenomyosis. *Int J Womens Health.* 2013 13; 5: 293-9.
[13] Maia Jr. H, Haddad C, Casoy J. Combining oral contraceptives with a natural nuclear factor-kappa B inhibitor for the treatment of endometriosis-related pain. *Int J Womens Health.* 2012; 21; 6: 35-9.
[14] Baskin GB, Smith SM, Marx PA. Endometrial hyperplasia, polyps and adenomyosis associated with unopposed estrogens in rhesus monkey (Macaca mulata). *Vet Pathol* 2002; 39:572-75.
[15] Maia H, Jr., Casoy J, Pimentel K, Correia T, Athayde C, Cruz T *et al.,* Effect of oral contraceptives on vascular endothelial growth factor, Cox-2 and aromatase expression in the endometrium of uteri affected by myomas and associated pathologies. *Contraception* 2008; 78: 479-85.
[16] McLucas B. Does endometrial resection cause adenomyosis? *J Am Assoc Gynecol Laparosc* 1994 1(4): S21.

[17] Hatok J, Zubor P, Galo S et al., Endometrial aromatase mRNA as a possible screening tool for advanced endometriosis and adenomyosis. *Gynecol Endocrinol* 2011:27(5): 331-6.

[18] Fechner S, Husen B, Thole H et al., Expression and regulation of estrogen converting enzymes in ectopic human endometrial tissue. *Fertil. Steril.* 2007; 88 (Suppl. 4): 1029–1038.

[19] Yamanak K, Xu B, Suganuma I et al., Dienogest inhibits aromatase and cyclooxygenase-2 expression and prostaglandin E2 production in human endometriotic stroma cells in spheroid cultures. *Fertil. Steril.* 2012; 97 (2), 477–482.

[20] Koike H, Egawa W, Ohtsuka T, Yamaguchi M, Ikenoue T, Mori N. Correlation between dysmenorrheic severity and prostaglandin production in women with endometriosis. *Prostaglandins Leukot Essent Fatty Acids* 1992; 46, 133–137.

[21] Maia Jr. H, Haddad C , Pinheiro N , Casoy J. Advantages of the association of resveratrol with oral contraceptives for management of endometriosis-related pain. *Int J Women's Health* 2012; 4: 543-9.

[22] Howe LR, Subbaramaiah K, Hudis CA, Dannenberg AJ. Molecular pathways: adipose inflammation as a mediator of obesity-associated cancer. *Clin Can Res* 2013 :19 (22): 6074-83.

[23] Bulun SE, Zeitoun K, Takayama K, Noble L, Michael D, Simpson E, Johns A,Putman M, Sasano H. Estrogen production in endometriosis and use of aromatase inhibitors to treat endometriosis. *Endocr Relat Cancer.* 1999 Jun;6 (2): 293-301.

[24] Mints M, Blomgren B, Palmblad J. Expression of vascular endothelial growth factor receptor-3 in the endometrium in menorrhagia. *Int J Mol Med.* 2007 Jun;19(6):909-13.

[25] Mints M, Hultenby K, Zetterberg E, Blomgren B, Falconer C, Rogers R, Palmblad J. Wall discontinuities and increased expression of vascular endothelial growth factor-A and vascular endothelial growth factor receptors 1 and 2 in endometrial blood vessels of women with menorrhagia. *Fertil Steril.* 2007 Sep;88 (3): 691-7.

[26] Saliou C, Rimbach G, Moini H, McLaughlin L, Hosseini S, Lee J, Watson RR, Packer L. Solar ultraviolet-induced erythema in human skin and nuclear factor-kappa-B-dependent gene expression in keratinocytes are modulated by a French maritime pine bark extract. *Free Radic Biol Med.* 2001 Jan 15;30 (2): 154-60.

[27] Wang Y, Lee KW, Chan FL, Chen S, Leung LK. The red wine polyphenol resveratrol displays bilevel inhibition on aromatase in breast cancer cells. *Toxicol Sci.* 2006 Jul;92 (1): 71-7.

[28] Zheng X, Zhu S, Chang S, Cao Y, Dong J, Li J, Long R, Zhou Y. Protective effects of chronic resveratrol treatment on vascular inflammatory injury in streptozotocin-induced type 2 diabetic rats: role of NF-kappa B signaling. *Eur J Pharmacol.* 2013;720(1-3):147-57.

[29] Wang Y, Leung LK. Pharmacological concentration of resveratrol suppresses aromatase in JEG-3 cells. *Toxicol Lett.* 2007 Sep 28;173(3):175-80.

[30] Chávez E, Reyes-Gordillo K, Segovia J, Shibayama M, Tsutsumi V, Vergara P, Moreno MG, Muriel P. Resveratrol prevents fibrosis *Am J Physiol Heart Circ Physiol.* 2006 Oct;291(4):H1694-9.

[31] Di Donato N, Montanari G, Benfenati A, Leonardi D, Bertoldo V, Monti G, Raimondo D, Seracchioli R. Prevalence of adenomyosis in women undergoing surgery for endometriosis. *N Eur J Obstet Gynecol Reprod Biol.* 2014 Oct;181: 289-93.

[32] Coutinho EM, Azadian--Boulanger G. Treatment of endometriosis by vaginal administration of gestrinone. *Fertil Steril.* 1988: 49(3): 418--22.

[33] Coutinho E, Gonçalves MT, Azadian--Boulanger G, Silva AR. Endometriosis therapy with gestrinone by oral, vaginal or parental administration. *Contr. Gynec. Obstet.* 1987; 16: 227-- 235.

[34] Dominique De Ziegler, Carlo Bulletti, Béatrice de Monstier and Anna--Stina Jääskeläinen. (1997) The First Uterine Pass Effect. The Uterus: Endometrium and Myometrium, *Annals of the New York Academy of Sciences.*

[35] Maia Jr. H, Haddad C, Casoy J. The effect of a combination of vaginal danazol with pycnogenol on pelvic pain in patients with deep endometriosis using Mirena. *Europ. J. Contracept. Reprod. Health Care:* 2014; 19 (Suppl 1, 208).

[36] Iwasaki Y, Asai M, Yoshida M, Nigawara T, Kambayashi M, Nakashima N. Dehydroepiandrosterone-sulfate inhibits nuclear factor-kappaB-dependent transcription in hepatocytes, possibly through antioxidant effect. *J Clin Endocrinol Metab.* 2004 Jul; 8 9(7): 3449-54.

In: Menorrhagia and Dysmenorrhea
Editor: Timothy M. Welch
ISBN: 978-1-63482-552-8

Chapter IV

Management of Dysmenorrhea in Women with Endometriosis

Ilaria Erasmo and Simone Ferrero*
IRCCS San Martino Hospital and National Institute for Cancer Research,
University of Genoa, Italy

Abstract

Dysmenorrhea is the most symptoms in women with endometriosis; its intensity is often severe and causes a significant decrease in quality of life. It is often associated with other pain symptoms (such as deep dyspareunia, dyschezia, non-menstrual pelvic pain). The pathogenesis of dysmenorrhea in women with endometriosis remains uncertain; it may be due to nociceptive, inflammatory and neuropathic mechanisms. Two types of therapy for endometriosis-related dysmenorrhea are available: pharmacological therapies that inhibit the growth of the endometriotic implants and surgical therapies, which aim to remove the endometriotic implants. Various hormonal treatments have been shown to effectively and safely relieve pain: non-steroidal anti-inflammatory drugs, progestins, androgens, combined oral contraceptive pill, gonadotropin

* Corresponding author: Simone Ferrero, MD, PhD, Department of Obstetrics and Gynecology, San Martino Hospital and National Institute for Cancer Research, University of Genoa, Italy, Largo R. Benzi 1, 16132, Genova, Italy, E-mail: simone.ferrero@unige.it, Telephone: 01139 010511525, Fax: 01139 010511525.

releasing hormones analogues, gonadotropin releasing hormones antagonists and aromatase inhibitors. Hormonal therapies do not cure endometriosis, therefore patients require a long-term treatment. All hormonal therapies are contraceptive and, therefore, they cannot be administered to patients desiring to conceive. Given this background, the choice of the drug should be based on the preference of the patients, on the incidence of adverse effects and on costs. Surgical excision of endometriosis is a valuable option in patients with severe dysmenorrhea desiring to conceive, in those who have persistence of the symptom despite the administration of hormonal therapies and in those who have contraindications to the use of hormonal therapies. However, dysmenorrhea may recur after surgery if patients do not receive a post-operative hormonal therapy.

Introduction

Dysmenorrhea is defined as pain associated with menstruation. This symptom is characterized by abdominal cramping in the lower abdomen, in the suprapubic region, and it may radiate to the thighs and lower back. It may occur before and during menstruation and may interfere with daily activity. Related general symptoms, such as nausea, vomiting, diarrhea and headache, are frequent [Harada, 2013]. Pain may be exacerbated by physical activity [Giudice, 2010].

The prevalence of dysmenorrhea ranges from 45% to 95% in developed countries and it is even more widespread in adolescent girls [Chang et al., 2012]. In the USA, 30% to 50% of women of childbearing age suffer from moderate to severe dysmenorrhea, and 10% to 20% of them suffer from severe pain and cannot lead a normal life [Jeon et al., 2014].

Dysmenorrhea is classified as primary and secondary. In primary dysmenorrhea, there is no underlying pelvic pathology; in contrast, secondary dysmenorrhea refers to menstrual pain due to an underlying pathology [Harada, 2013].

Secondary dysmenorrhea appears more than 5 years after menarche, over 30 years old, became worst and has a duration of 1 to 5 days and it can persist beyond menses; while primary dysmenorrhea arise in younger age (15-25 years old), usually improves with aging and has a duration of 4 to 48 hours [Harada, 2013]. The most common cause of secondary dysmenorrhea is endometriosis [Harada, 2013].

Epidemiology of Dysmenorrhea in Women with Endometriosis

Women with endometriosis have a high prevalence of dysmenorrhea, and the presence of this symptom has been demonstrated to be a suggestive predictor of endometriosis [Whitehill et al., 2012]. Actually the hypothesis is that a large number of patients who are suffering from dysmenorrhea have endometriosis [Hansen et al., 2013].

In patients suffering from dysmenorrhea, the incidence of endometriosis ranges from 40% to 60% and the 70% of adolescents who experience dysmenorrhea are diagnosed with endometriosis [Propst et al., 1999].

In patients with endometriosis dysmenorrhea is often associated with other pain symptoms including non-menstrual pelvic pain, deep dyspareunia and dyschezia. These patients may also suffer urinary and intestinal symptoms when endometriosis involves the bladder and the bowel, respectively.

Pathogenesis of Dysmenorrhea in Women with Endometriosis

The mechanism by which endometriosis causes dysmenorrhea remains uncertain [Howard, 2009]. Pain may be due to nociceptive, inflammatory and neuropathic mechanisms. There is no precise relationship between the severity of the disease and the intensity of dysmenorrhea [Howard, 2009].

Nociceptive pain may have both somatic and visceral origin. Pain due to endometriosis is visceral in origin because endometriosis affects both pelvic viscera and visceral peritoneum. Nociceptors are present in the uterus and cervix, this evidence is based on electrophysiological recordings [Berkley et al., 1990] and on the immunocyto-chemical labeling of substance P and calcitonin gene-related peptide in uterine nerve fibers [Tong et al., 2006].

Some nociceptors in viscera are "silent nociceptors"; in fact, they physiologically do not respond to mechanical or thermal stimuli, but they become sensitized and will respond to these stimuli when inflammation is present in the tissue [Gebhart et al., 2000]. Actually it has been shown that endometriosis changes the population of uterine nociceptors and stimulates an abnormal presence of nociceptors in or near peritoneal endometriotic lesions [Howard, 2009]. There are evidences that endometriosis can behave as a noxious stimulus and trigger transduction [Howard, 2009]. The existence of neuropathic pain in endometriosis is supported by various clinical trials of laparoscopic surgical ablation or excision of endometriosis: when endometriosis, that is considerate the noxious stimulus, is removed, the pain should finish [Sutton et al., 1994; Abbot et al., 2004].

Inflammation is very important in visceral pain [Howard, 2009]. Endometriosis is characterized by aberrant immuno-inflammatory phenomena. Near the endometriotic lesions, in uterine endometrium and in the peritoneal fluid of women with endometriosis there are high levels of inflammatory factors (immune cells and pro-inflammatory mediators which present an altered function). Lymphocytes and particularly activated macrophages secrete growth factors and pro-inflammatory cytokines, and thus they maintain the inflammatory response [Howard, 2009].

Prostaglandins (PGs) are major immuno-inflammatory mediators and are involved in dysmenorrhea. The normal endometrium produces prostaglandins; in endometriotic lesions there are differences in the production of PGs that is under the control of ovarian hormones [Olavi et al., 1983]. Estrogen and progesterone receptors are present in endometriotic implants that respond to variations of hormonal levels with bleeding or release of inflammatory products, particularly prostaglandins E_2 (PGE_2) and prostaglandin F (PGF) [Howard, 2009]. PGE_2 and PGF are direct generators of pain because they activate nerve endings to pain and induce the release of histamine, serotonin, nerve growth factor, prostanoids and others algesic mediators [Howard, 2009]. Women with endometriosis have more peritoneal macrophages than women without the disease and these macrophages secrete an increased quantity of PGE_2 and PGF2α [Karck et al., 1996], and they also have a higher concentration of PGE_2 and PGF2α in their eutopic endometrium or peritoneal fluid [Weed, 1980; William et al., 1976]. The higher level of PGE_2 is due to the up-regulation of the Cox-2 isoenzyme; indeed PGs in endometriosis are produced by this enzyme [Matsuzaki et al., 2004]. It is demonstrated that there is an increased level of this enzyme in the epithelium and stroma of endometriosis compared with normal endometrium of patients without the disease, and that its levels are also higher in eutopic endometrium of women with endometriosis than in the endometrium obtained from controls. There is a positive feedback loop that causes the incessant synthesis of estradiol and PGE_2 in endometriosis, thus PGE_2 is the most effective of the stimulators of the steroidogenic acute regulatory proteins and aromatase, that are present in endometriotic implants and that induce the synthesis of estradiol [Giudice et al., 2004; Koike et al., 1992].

In both endometriosis and dysmenorrhea there are abnormal patterns of uterine contractility [Dawood, 1990]. Characteristics of uterine contraction during menses vary in women with mild to moderate endometriosis and in healthy women. Bulletti et al., [Bulletti et al., 2002] performed a controlled prospective study to assess the frequency, amplitude, and basal pressure tone of uterine contractions and correlation of contractions with retrograde bleeding and presence of viable endometrial cells and dysmenorrhea before and 3 and 24 months after surgery for infertility in women with and without endometriosis. They found that myometrial activity was increased in women with endometriosis and that in presence of the disease, basal pressure tone, frequency of uterine contractions, and amplitude and incidence of retrograde contractions were higher. This study demonstrated that dyskinetic alterations of uterine contractility during menses play a role in the process of endometriosis [Bulletti et al., 2002]. Prostaglandins are of paramount importance in the regulation of normal and abnormal uterine activity, above all during menstruation. Uterus performs a particular pattern of natural activity that fluctuates according to the different phases of the menstrual cycle. This different pattern of contractility depend on variation in estrogen and progesterone levels, but prostaglandins are also involved; in particular $PGF_2\alpha$ regulates the normal uterine activity but it is also important for the appearance of pathological motility [Bygdeman et al., 1979].

Nerve Growth Factors (NGF) has been recently proposed as one of the factors that have a causative role in pain. NGF is locally produced in endometriotic lesions. Positive immunoreactivity for NGF has been shown near the endometrial glands in peritoneal endometriotic lesions, and in ovarian and rectovaginal endometriosis [Kajitani et al., 2013]. NGF has the capacity to attract mast cells and to cause their degranulation, thus this humoral factor has the ability to maintain persistent inflammatory pain.

Deeply infiltrating lesions (DIE), which consistently cause pelvic pain and is a infiltrating > 5 mm, contains more activated mast cells than peritoneal and ovarian lesions, which are less substantial sources of pain.

Mast cells are present in higher quantity in DIE in proximity with nerves than in peritoneal and ovarian endometriosis [Anaf et al., 2006]. Mast cells probably play a role in the development of fibrosis and adhesions and they are also involved in the occurrence of pelvic pain [Morotti et al., 2014a]. Women with severe dysmenorrhea present a higher quantity of nerve fibers within the endometriotic nodules and a closer histological relationship between the nerve fibers, fibrosis and endometriotic nodules is present in these patients [Anaf et al., 2006].

Neural plasticity and central sensitization have a critical role in neuropathic pain [Howard, 2009]. The differences in endometrial nerve fibers density and quality in women with endometriosis makes pain associated with endometriosis easy to understand. Severity of pain correlates with the depth of infiltration into peritoneum or pelvic organs and the pro-inflammatory products released by the implants or neighboring tissues into peritoneal fluid [Morotti et al., 2014a]. Various studies suggest that there is a mechanism of neuroangiogenesis in endometriosis [Mechsner et al., 2007; Mechsner et al., 2009; Tokushige et al., 2006].

Is currently known the possibility of central sensitization in patients with endometriosis related pain. This dysfunction of the central nervous system unfolds with hyper excitability and sensitization. It is demonstrated that in women who suffer from chronic pelvic pain there are significant central changes and these changes may exacerbate the pain [Brawn et al., 2014].

Treatment of Dysmenorrhea

Two types of therapy for endometriosis-related dysmenorrhea are available: pharmacological therapies that inhibit the growth of the endometriotic implants, and surgical therapies, which aim to remove the endometriotic implants. A combined medical and conservative surgical approach brings benefit to many women with endometriosis-associated pain. The surgical excision of endometriotic lesions causes improvement of dysmenorrhea, but this symptom may recur after surgery. Medical treatment may be used to treat recurrent symptoms or prevent recurrence of endometriosis.

Hormonal Treatment

Endometriosis is estrogen dependent, thus medical therapies are focused on reducing estrogen levels. Various hormonal treatments have been shown to effectively and safely relieve pain: non-steroidal anti-inflammatory drugs (NSAIDs), progestins, androgens (danazol), combined oral contraceptive pill (COC), gonadotropin releasing hormones analogues (GnRH-a), gonadotropin releasing hormones antagonists (GnRH-ant), and aromatase inhibitors (AIs).

Non-Steroidal Anti-Inflammatory Drugs

NSAIDs are the first line-treatment for dysmenorrhea due to endometriosis and they are a fundamental option for women who attempting to conceive [Ferrero et al., 2010a]. NSAIDs inhibit the cyclooxygenase (COX) enzymes and so the production of Pgs. Recent studies demonstrated that indometacin diminishes the growth of endometriotic cysts and restores fertility in the rat model of endometriosis; rofecoxib causes the regression and atrophy of endometriotic lesions. However, these preliminary observations remain to be confirmed in humans [Ferrero et al., 2010a]. NSAIDs are the most common used drugs because they have few side effects in low dose; however, women using NSAIDs need to be aware of the possibility that these drugs may cause unintended effects in high dose (increased risk of gastrointestinal and nervous system adverse effect) [Allen et al., 2009]. A recent Cochrane review demonstrated that NSAIDs are an effective treatment for pain caused by primary dysmenorrhea [Marjoribanks et al., 2003]. However, there isn't evidence to prove whether NSADs are effective for the treatment of pain caused by endometriosis and there isn't also evidence to indicate whether any individual NSAID is more effective than others [Marjoribanks et al., 2003].

Progestins

Several progestins have been employed in the hormonal treatment of endometriosis, as oral and injectable formulation; some of these drugs have been used as part of oral contraceptive combinations. The rationale for using progestin consists of the fact that they have anti-gonadotropic properties and enhance the negative feedback of estrogen at the hypothalamus causing hypo gonadotropic hypo-estrogenic anovulation. Thus endometriosis-related dysmenorrhea back off because of the amenorrhea. This treatment can be administered only to women who do not wish to conceive [Mehedintu et al., 2014]. However there is no evidence that the cyclical administration of progestin may improve dysmenorrhea or fertility. Unfortunately, dysmenorrhea recurs after cessation of treatment [Mehedintu et al., 2014]. Irregular uterine bleeding is the most common adverse effect that usually occurs in the long-term progestin treatments, so informing women of this common effect before they initiate treatment enhances the long-term adherence to therapy [Mehedintu et al., 2014].

Medroxyprogesterone acetate (MPA) has been used for many years for treating dysmenorrhea caused by endometriosis. It can be administered orally in doses between 30 and 50 mg/day, by intramuscular injections or subcutaneously. In two randomized controlled trials (RCTs), Telimaa et al., demonstrated that the administration of MPA (100 mg/day) for 6 months is as effective as danazol in the treatment of endometriosis-related pain both after diagnostic laparoscopy [Telimaa et al., 1987a] and after surgical excision of endometriosis [Telimaa et al., 1987b]. One prospective double-blind RCT involving 48 women with surgical diagnosis of endometriosis compared MPA and GnRH-a in the treatment of pain symptoms caused by endometriosis [Bergqvist et al., 2001]. Patients were treated for 6 months and followed for 1 year after allocation. There was a significant reduction in the severity of pain symptoms during the study, without any significant difference between the study groups. However these results are in contrast to a prospective, double-blind RCT involving 100 infertile women with surgical diagnosis of endometriosis, which compared the efficacy of 3-month administration of MPA (50 mg/day) with placebo [Harrison et al., 2000]. In this study MPA and placebo were equally effective in decreasing pain and the American Fertility Society scores of endometriosis at second-look laparoscopy. However, the short length of treatment is an important limitation and may have biased the results [Ferrero et al., 2010a]. The oral administration of MPA presents disadvantages including the need for strict daily compliance, the variable absorption from the gastrointestinal tract, and the peaks and troughs associated with the short half-lives of the preparation. The use of a depot preparation of MPA (DMPA) administered intramuscularly eliminates these problems.

A RCT compared the treatment for 1 year with intramuscular DMPA (150 mg every 3 months) with a cyclic monophasic oral contraceptive combined with very low dose oral danazol (50 mg/day for 21 days of each 28-day cycle) [Vercellini et al., 1996]. A decrease was observed in the intensity of all pain symptoms with no differences between the study groups. At the 1-year, 72.5% of the patients receiving DMPA were satisfied, compared with 57.5% of those receiving the double-drug regimen. A significant decrease of high-density lipoprotein (HDL) and cholesterol occurred in both the study groups. Breakthrough bleeding or spotting was observed in 80% of patients treated with DMPA and in 10% of control women. Actually a new subcutaneous preparation of DMPA has been formulated. Two multicenter, 18-month, evaluator-blinded RCTs involving patients with surgical diagnosis of endometriosis compared the subcutaneous formulation of DMPA (104 mg/0.65 ml every 3 months) with the long-acting depot preparation of leuprolide acetate in the treatment of endometriosis-related pain symptoms [Crosignani et al., 2006; Schlaff et al., 2006]. Treatments caused amenorrhea and they were equally effective in treating the other pain symptoms; however,

DMPA caused a lower bone mineral density decline, fewer hypo-estrogenic adverse effects and more frequent episodes of uterine bleeding.

Norethisterone acetate (or norethindrone acetate, NETA) is a 19-nortestosterone derivative. An oral dosage between 5 and 20 mg per day significantly improves dysmenorrhea in women with surgical diagnosis of endometriosis. Vercellini et al., in a prospective RCT, confronted the effectiveness of a 12-month course of NETA (2.5 mg daily) with a COC containing ethinylestradiol (0.01 mg) and cyproterone acetate (3 mg/day). This study involved 90 patient suffering from severe or moderate pain due to endometriosis who before underwent conservative surgery for recto-vaginal endometriosis. After twelve months of continuous therapy, similar improvement in symptoms score was noted in both groups. Only 7 women (16%) in the COC group and 5 (11%) in the NETA group experienced important adverse effects or persistent pain and thereby interrupted the treatment [Vercellini et al., 2005]. NETA consent good control of uterine bleeding, it presents positive effects on calcium metabolism and it hasn't important negative effects on the lipoprotein metabolism when used at low dose, thus it is suitable for the long-term treatment of endometriosis-related pain [Vercellini et al., 2003a].

Cyproterone acetate (CPA) is a derivate of 17α-idrossi progesterone with anti-androgenic and anti-gonadotropic properties. It has been combined with ethinylestradiol as an oral contraceptive, but has also used as monotherapy for the treatment of endometriosis [Ferrero et al., 2010a]. In 1996, Moran et al., evaluated the efficacy of 6-month treatment with CPA (10 mg/day for 20 days followed by 10 days with no treatment) in seven women with mild to severe symptomatic endometriosis. Dysmenorrhea was relieved significantly in all of the patients. At the end of treatment a second look laparoscopy noted minimal endometriosis in five patients and no evidence of the disease in the other two cases. These findings encouraged the use of CPA in the treatment of endometriosis [Moran et al., 1996]. A RCT examined CPA monotherapy for pain related to endometriosis. This RCT involved 90 women suffer from recurrent pelvic pain after a conservative surgical treatment. Patients were randomized to receive either CPA (12.5 mg per day) or an OCP (ethinylestradiol 0.02 mg and desogestrel 0.15 mg). Important and analogue improvements in symptoms were assessed in both groups. 73% of women in the CPA group and the 67% those in the COC group were satisfied with the treatment received.

Desogestrel (DSG) is a third-generation progestin that is used for hormonal contraception alone and also as oral contraceptive [Scala et al.,

2013]. It has been used in the treatment of endometriosis both as primary therapy [Ferrero et al., 2013] and as an adjunct to surgical resection [Razzi et al., 2007]. A RCT demonstrated that both DSG and OCP decrease the intensity of dysmenorrhea after conservative surgery [Razzi et al., 2007]. A 12-month management with DSG reduced the size of rectovaginal endometriotic nodules [Ferrero et al., 2013].

Dienogest (DNG) is a derivative of 19-nortestosterone that juxtapose the pharmacological properties of 19-nortestosterone derivatives (such as the short plasma half-life, the powerful progestin effect on the endometrium and the high bioavailability) with those of natural progesterone derivatives (such as moderate inhibition of gonadotropin secretion and anti-androgenic activity). DNG has high selectivity for the progesteron receptors and a powerful progestinic effect on the endometrium [Bizzarri et al., 2014]. The efficacy of DNG in the treatment of endometriosis may depend on its capacity to determinate a hypo-estrogenic and hyper-progestinic endocrine environment, which, at first, causes the decidualization of ectopic endometrial tissue, but for prolonged therapies, DNG determines atrophy of the endometriotic lesions. A multicenter RCT confronted the effectiveness of DNG (2 mg/day for 12 weeks) with placebo; DNG was significantly more effective than placebo in reducing endometriosis associated pelvic pain [Strowitzki et al., 2010a]. Women who participated at this 12-week study were offered the possibility to enter an open-label extension study of DNG for up to 53 additional weeks, providing an overall treatment period of up to 65 weeks. A high number (n =168, 89%) of the 188 women completing the placebo-controlled study, agreed to enter the long-term extension study. The intensity of pain demonstrated remarkable improvements during the long-term study, in addition to those caused by DNG during the first phase of the study [Strowitzki et al., 2010a]. During a 24-week treatment-free period following the long-term study, pain scores increased but mildly. This fact may show that DNG determines a positive effect that persists after treatment cessation; indeed the drugs may have multiple mechanisms of action which decreased the growth and the neoangiogenesis of the lesions and provides an anti-inflammatory effect. Another explanation for this long-term effect is the decrease of endometriotic lesions during DNG therapy [Petraglia et al., 2011]. Adverse effects occurred in 16.1% of patients; they included breast discomfort (4.2%), nausea (3.0%) and irritability (2.4%). The maximal intensity of treatment- related adverse events was mild or moderate in 92.5% of cases. During the long-term study the intensity and frequency of bleeding decreased and during follow-up, bleeding returned to normal intensity and cyclic patterns resumed within 4-6 weeks. Treatment compliance during the long-term study was 98% and discontinuation rates due to adverse events or lack of efficacy were both low (2.4% and 0.6%, respectively) [Strowitzki et al., 2010a].

Recent trials compared DNG with GnRH-a. One of these trials was a 24-week, multicenter, randomized, open-label, parallel-group study of DNG versus leuprolide acetate (LA). Patients were randomized to receive DNG (2 mg orally once daily) or LA (3.75 mg as a depot i.m. injection every 4 weeks). This study included 252 women with endometriosis diagnosed by laparoscopy. DNG and LA led to a continuous and comparable reduction of pelvic pain. At the end of the 24 weeks, the reduction in the average VAS score was 47.5 mm for the DNG group and 46 mm for the LA group; this study demonstrated that DNG isn't inferior compared with LA and that compared with LA, which presents hypo estrogenic effects that limit long-term use, DNG was associated with a safety profile in this trial [Strowitzki et al., 2010b]. A recent study assesses the management of DNG in a pre-treated NETA sample: in this study DNG (2 mg/day) caused significant improvements in endometriosis associated-pain, with a safety and tolerability profile. It was demonstrated the efficacy of DNG in treating women with pain symptoms“resistant” to NETA [Morotti et al., 2014b].

The role of a long-acting, locally administered progestin in the form of medicated intrauterine device (Lng-IUD) has recently considered an interesting treatment. The Lng-IUD is an option of hormonal treatment with a progestin, which locally produces therapeutic concentrations and also has few systemic side effects. The Lng-IUD diminishes the intensity of dysmenorrhea and the size of endometriotic implants in patients with rectovaginal endometriosis. [Fedele et al., 2001].

A prospective non-comparative observational study showed that the Lng-IUD improves endometriosis-related dysmenorrhea; in this study 34 women with minimal to moderate endometriosis had Lng-IUS inserted for 6 months. The intensity of dysmenorrhea decreased and there was a reduction in the frequency of pain (id est. number of days of pain per month). The extension of the endometriotic lesions observed at a second look laparoscopy improved [Lockhat et al., 2004]. Vercellini et al., assessed the effectiveness of Lng-IUD in preventing the recurrence of symptoms after conservative surgery for endometriosis; the authors shown that the frequency and severity of dysmenorrhea were decreased in women treated with Lng-IUD after operative laparoscopy compared with patients treated only with surgery [Vercellini et al., 2003b].

The etonogestrel subdermal implant (EngSI) is a single ethylene vinyl acetate copolymer rod containing 68 mg etonogestrel (3-ketodesogestrel). It has contraceptive efficacy for 3 years because it inhibits ovulation, determines endometrial suppression, alters cervical mucus that become inadequate and causes an abnormal luteal phase. A RCT compared the therapeutic efficacy of the EngSI with DMPA. The improvement of pain was comparable for the two therapies. The adverse effects profile observed in EngSI users was similar to that observed in DMPA users. An unintentional weight gain of more than 10% of the baseline weight was experienced in 9.5% of women in the EngSI group and in 20% of patients in the DMPA group. Thus in patients with high body mass index EngSI could be preferable to DMPA. Lately the EngSI has been used with Lng-IUD to treat pelvic pain due to endometriosis not responding to others treatments [Walch et al., 2009].

The long-term treatment with progestin may have negative influence on bone mineral density [Beerthuizen et al., 2000]. In an open, prospective, comparative study, the effect of the EngSI on BMD was compared to a non-hormone-medicated intrauterine device (IUD). Changes of BMD in the EngSI group were not different from those in the IUD group. The Eng-SI may be an additional innovative, effective, safe, well-tolerated and convenient long-term treatment option in women with symptomatic endometriosis who also need contraception [Affandi, 1998].

Danazol

Danazol is an isoxazol derivative of 17α-ethinyl testosterone; it was the first drug to be approved for the treatment of endometriosis in the US. Danazol produces a high androgen and low estrogen environment, which results in the atrophy of the endometriotic implants and so in the improvement of pain symptoms [Selak et al., 2007]. However, danazol causes significant androgenic adverse effects (for example hair growth and mood changes) and, therefore, the use of this this drugs for the long-term treatment of endometriosis is not recommended.

Combined Oral Contraceptives

COC have been used empirically to relieve dysmenorrhea for many years. The long-term therapy with COC is generally easily acceptable and thus they are frequently administered to women with endometriosis related dysmenorrhea. A double-blind RCT evaluated the efficacy of low-dose COC for patients with dysmenorrhea associated with endometriosis. This study demonstrated for the first time that low-dose OCPs decrease the intensity of dysmenorrhea associated with endometriosis compared with placebo. COC reduced the days analgesics were used and improved the quality of life in these women [Harada et al., 2011]. Continuous COC treatment may be more effective than cyclic treatment. In women with endometriosis-associated recurrent dysmenorrhea that does not respond to cyclic COC use, a long-term reduction of pain symptoms and an important degree of satisfaction with treatment can be achieved by continuous therapy with COC [Vercellini et al., 2003c]. A 12-month administration of COC determines a decrease in the size of rectovaginal endometriotic nodules [Ferrero et al., 2013]. Estroprogestin combinations in the non-oral forms (contraceptive patch, contraceptive vaginal ring) have also been prescribed to treat endometriosis-related dysmenorrhea.

Gonadotrophin Releasing Hormone Analogues

One of the primary medications used in the treatment of endometriosis were GnRH-a. They are modified forms of GnRH that bind to receptors in the pituitary gland and have longer half-life than native GnRH. The agonistic effect is an initial stimulation, which is followed by suppression of gonadotropins; therefore, these agents rapidly induce a hypo-estrogenic state similar to that of menopause, producing progressive endometrial atrophy and amenorrhea. GnRH-a can be administered by a nasal spray or by injection of either a short-acting formulation daily or a depot formulation (every 1 or 3 months). A double-blind RCT involving 49 women compared the effects on pain symptoms of 6-month treatment with GnRH-a (triptorelin) or placebo. The study showed that triptorelin effectively decreases the intensity of pain symptoms caused by endometriosis [Bergqvist et al., 1998]. GnRH-an and danazol are equivalent in the treatment of the dysmenorrhea. [Prentice et al., 2000]. Other RCTs demonstrated that GnRH-a are as effective as MPA [Bergqvist et al., 2001] and the Lng-IUD [Petta et al., 2005] in treating pain symptoms caused by endometriosis. A systematic review found that GnRH-a are more effective than low-dose monophasic COC in the treatment of dysmenorrhea [Davis et al., 2007]. Another RCT compared COC given for 12 months and GnRH-a given for 4 months followed by COC treatment for 8 months in the relief of endometriosis-related pain. At 1-year follow-up, the two treatments showed similar relief of pain symptoms [Parazzini et al., 2000]. In addition, the administration of GnRH-a after surgical treatment prolongs the pain-free interval and postpones the requirement of further treatment [Hornstein et al., 1997]. The major limitation of the long-term treatment with GnRH-a is the incidence of adverse effects cause by the hypoestrogenic state. These adverse effects include hot flashes, insomnia, reduction in bone mineral density, vaginal dryness, decreased libido, depression, joint pain, mood swings and fatigue [Prentice et al., 2000]. The adverse effects of GnRH-a can be ameliorated by the administration of add-back therapies, which include a progestin only, a progestin plus bisphosphonate or a progestin plus estrogen. A 1-year, double-blind RCT involving 201 women with endometriosis treated with GnRH analogues reported improvement in pain symptoms and preservation of bone mineral density in patients receiving progestin only (NETA 5 mg daily) or progestin (NETA 5 mg daily) plus conjugated equine oestrogen (0.625 mg daily) [Hornstein et al., 1998].

Gonadotrophin Releasing Hormone Antagonist

GnRH-ant have recently been introduced in the treatment of endometriosis. These drugs decrease estrogen levels but they do not cause the side effects related to estrogen deprivation. Furthermore, GnRH-ant does not cause the initial gonadotropic peak because they do not cause the stimulation of the pituitary-ovarian axis. A recent randomized double-blind study demonstrated that elagolix, a short-acting, GnRH-ant, administered orally, has the potential to become a new treatment option for the management of endometriosis associated pain. This GnRH-ant has a short half-life (~6 hours) and a rapid elimination from the body. Elagolix was statistically non-inferior to DMPA, for reducing the dysmenorrhea related to endometriosis. The tolerability of elagolix and DMPA was similar. Patients treated with elagolix manifested a higher reduction in uterine bleeding. Overall, there was a high rate of hot flashes in all groups [Diamond et al., 2014].

Aromatase Inhibitors

Several studies in the past have demonstrated that aromatase P450 is over-expressed in eutopic but also in ectopic endometrium of patients with endometriosis and that it is not measurable in eutopic endometrium of healthy women and in endometriosis free peritoneal tissue [Ferrero et al., 2011; Ferrero et al., 2010b]. Third-generation AIs (letrozole and anastrozole) were used to treat pain symptoms in women with endometriosis. AIs inhibit the enzyme catalyzing the main step of the estrogen synthesis. In premenopausal women, they stimulate ovarian function because they causes the decrease in circulating estrogens and thus the increase of the gonadotropin secretion; for this reason the continuous management of AIs in reproductive age women with endometriosis must be combined with ovarian suppressive agents (such as the oral contraceptive pills or progestins). Studies demonstrated that AIs associated with either progestogens, oral contraceptive pill or gonadotropin releasing hormone analogue reduce the intensity of pain symptoms caused by endometriosis. However, pain symptoms usually recur after the discontinuation of treatment and, after 6 months from the end of therapy, the intensity of pain symptoms was about equal to pre-treatment values [Ferrero et al., 2009; Remorgida et al., 2007a; Remorgida et al., 2007b]. The management of AIs in premenopausal women may produce more severe adverse effects (such as arthralgia and myalgia) than those caused by progestins and COC thus reducing the compliance of the patients in the long-term treatment [Ferrero et al., 2011]. AIs may also have a role in the prevention of recurrence after surgical treatment of endometriosis. Because the administration of AIs to patients with endometriosis should be considered experimental, only patients failing to improve after the administration of standard hormonal therapies and surgical treatment are eligible to receive this therapy.

Surgical Treatment

Laparotomy and laparoscopy improve equally the endometriosis-associated dysmenorrhea, but laparoscopic surgery is typically followed by less pain, shorter hospital stay and quicker recovery as well as better cosmetic outcome, thus it is usually preferred to open surgery. The characteristics of the endometriotic implants vary the degree to which pain occurs. Deeply infiltrating endometriotic implants are most commonly associated with pain and superficial implants are often associated with minimal pain symptoms [Koninckx et al., 1991]. Laparoscopic excision of the lesions can be performed employing the ablative technique or the excision technique. A small RCT (24 women with pain caused by mild endometriosis) compared laparoscopic excision versus laparoscopic ablation of endometriotic lesions. The RCT found no differences between the two groups, with 67% of women in both treatment groups reporting good symptomatic relief [Wright et al., 2005]. A RCT including 39 women with stage I-IV endometriosis compared laparoscopic removal of endometriotic deposits alone (by excisional surgery) versus diagnostic laparoscopy in women with pain caused by endometriosis. Laparoscopic excision of endometriosis significantly improved pain symptoms compared with diagnostic laparoscopy at 6 months [Abbot et al., 2004]. Recurrence rate depend on the technique utilized, in particular for deep endometriosis. Rate of recurrence or persistence of endometriosis after ablation is approximately 20% to 50% in 2 years [Sutton et al., 1994] but as low as 0% at 2 years after optimal excision [Yeung et al., 2013]. Recurrence rate after conservative surgery, even for advanced or deep disease can be low (<10% in 3 years) [Vignali et al., 2005] and depends on the surgical completeness of removing the disease.

Radical surgical treatment may have to be explored in women suffering from dysmenorrhea related to endometriosis that is not achievable by medical and minor surgical intervention. Often, this involves the partial or complete removal of the reproductive organs (hysterectomy and/or oophorectomy). This option can be offered to women with chronic pelvic pain who completed their families and underwent other medical and or conservative surgical treatments. A potential reason to remove the uterus is the presence of adenomyosis.

Conclusion

The intensity of dysmenorrhea can be significantly improved by hormonal therapies and by surgery causing a significant amelioration in quality of life. The choice of the type of treatment (hormonal or surgical) should be based on the preference of the patients, the intensity of symptoms, the incidence of adverse effects and the cost of treatment. Surgical excision of endometriosis is a valuable option in patients with severe dysmenorrhea desiring to conceive, in those who have persistence of the symptom despite the administration of hormonal therapies and in those who have contraindications to the use of hormonal therapies. However, dysmenorrhea may recur after surgery and patients should be advised to undergo post-operative hormonal therapy. Progestins cause amenorrhea and, therefore, they are particularly useful in patients with endometriosis requiring treatment of dysmenorrhea. In addition, progestins cause less adverse effects than other therapies causing amenorrhea (such as GnRH-a) and are available in various formulations (oral tables, intrauterine device and subdermal implant.

References

Abbot, J; Hawe, J; Hunter, D; Holmes, M; Finn, P; Garry, R. Laparoscopic excision of endometriosis: a randomized placebo controlled trial. *Fertil Steril,* 2004 82(4), 878-884.

Affandi, B. An integrated analysis of vaginal bleeding patterns in clinical trials of Implanon. *Contraception,* 1998 58(6 Suppl), 99S-107S.

Allen, C; Hopewell, S; Prentice, A; Gregory, D. Non-steroidal anti-inflammatory drugs for pain in women with endometriosis. *Cochrane Database Syst. Rev.*, 2009 15(2), CD004753.

Anaf, V; Chapron, C; El Nakadi, I; De Moor, V; Simonart, T; Noel, JC. Pain, mast cells, and nerves in peritoneal, ovarian, and deep infiltrating endometriosis. *Fertil Steril*, 2006 86(5), 1336-1343.

Beerthuizen, R; Van Beek, A; Massai, R; Mäkäräinen, L; Hout, J; Bennink, HC. Bone mineral density during long-term use of the progestogen implant Implanon® compared to a non-hormonal method of contraception. *Hum. Reprod.*, 2000 15, 118–22.

Bergqvist, A; Bergh, T; Hogstrom, L; Mattsson, S; Nordenskjöld, F; Rasmussen, C. Effects of triptorelin versus placebo on the symptoms of endometriosis. *Fertil Steril*, 1998 69(4), 702-708.

Bergqvist, A; Theorell, T. Changes in quality of life after hormonal treatment of endometriosis. *Acta Obstet. Gynecol. Scand.*, 2001 80(7), 628-637.

Berkley, KJ; Hotta, H; Robbins, A; Sato, Y. Functional properties of afferent fibers supplying reproductive and other pelvic organs in pelvic nerve of female rat. *J Neurophysiol*, 1990 63(2), 256-272.

Bizzarri, N; Remorgida, V; Leone, Roberti, Maggiore, U; Scala, C; Tafi, E; Ghirardi, V; Salvatore, S; Candiani, M; Venturini, PL; Ferrero, S. Dienogest in the treatment of endometriosis. *Expert Opin Pharmacother*, 2014 15(13), 1889-1902.

Brawn, J; Morotti, M; Zondervan, KT; Becker, CM; Vincent, K. Central changes associated with chronic pelvic pain and endometriosis. *Hum. Reprod. Update*, 2014 20(5), 737-747.

Bulletti, C; De Ziegler, D; Polli, V; Del Ferro, E; Palini, S; Flamigni, C. Characteristics of uterine contractility during menses in women with mild to moderate endometriosis. *Fertil Steril*, 2002 77(6), 1156-1161.

Bygdeman, M; Bremme, K; Gillespie, A; Lundstrom, V. Effects of the prostaglandins on the uterus. *Acta Obset Gynaecol Scand Suppl*, 1979 87, 33-38.

Chang, SF; Chuang, M. Factors that affect self-care behaviour of female high school students with dysmenorrhoea: a cluster sampling study. *Int. J. Nurs. Pract.*, 2012 18(2), 117-124.

Crosignani, PG; Luciano, A; Ray A; Bergqvist, A. Subcutaneous depot medroxyprogesterone acetate versus leuprolide acetate in the treatment of endometriosis-associated pain. *Hum. Reprod.*, 2006 21(1), 248-256.

Davis, L; Kennedy, SS; Moore, J; Prentice, A; Modern combined oral contraceptives for pain associated with endometriosis. *Cochrane Database Syst. Rev.*, 2007 18(3), CD001019.

Dawood, MY.Dysmenorrhea. *Clin. Obstet. Gynecol.*, 1990 33(1), 168–178.

Diamond, MP; Carr, B; Dmowski, WP; Koltun, W; O'Brien, C; Jiang, P; Burke, J; Jimenez, R; Garner, E; Chwalisz, K. Elagolix treatment for endometriosis-associated pain: result from a phase 2, randomized, double blinde, placebo-controlled study. *Reproductive Scienzes*, 2014 21(3), 363-371.

Fedele, L; Bianchi, S; Zanconato, G; Portuese, A; Raffaelli R. Use of a levonorgestrel-releasing intrauterine device in the treatment of rectovaginal endometriosis. *Fertil Steril*, 2001 75(3), 485-488.

Ferrero, S; Camerini, G; Seracchioli, R; Ragni, N; Venturini, PL; Remorgida, V. Letrozole combined with norethisterone acetate compared with norethisterone acetate alone in the treatment of pain symptoms caused by endometriosis. *Hum. Reprod.*, 2009 24(12), 3033-3041.

Ferrero, S; Gillott, DJ; Venturini, PL; Remorgida, V. Use of aromatase inhibitors to treat endometriosis-related pain symptoms: a systematic review. *Reprod. Biol. Endocrinol.*, 2011 21(9), 89.

Ferrero, S; Leone, Roberti, Maggiore, U; Scala, C; Di Luca, M; Remorgida, V. Changes in the size of rectovaginal endometriotic nodules infiltrating the rectum during hormonal therapies. *Arch. Gynecol. Obstet.*, 2013 287(3), 447-453.

Ferrero, S; Remorgida, V; Venturini, PL. Current pharmacotherapy for endometriosis. *Expert Opin Pharmacother*, 2010a 11(7), 1123-1134.

Ferrero, S; Remorgida, V; Venturini, PL. Aromatase inhibitors in the treatment of endometriosis. In Endometriosis: Symptoms, Diagnosis and Treatments. Edited by: Mitchell LA. Nova Publishers, 2010b 213-224.

Gebhart, GF. J Bonica Lecture-2000: Physiology, pathophysiology, and pharmacology of visceral pain. *Reg. Anesth Pain Med.*, 2000 25(6), 632-638.

Giudice, LC. Clinical practice. Endometriosis. *N. Engl. J. Med.*, 2010 362(25), 2389-2398.

Giudice, LC; Kao, LC. Endometriosis. Lancet, 2004 364(9447), 1789–1799.

Hansen, SO; Knudsen, UB. Endometriosis, dysmenorrhoea and diet. *Eur. J. Obstet. Gynecol. Reprod. Biol.*, 2013 169(2), 162-171.

Harada, T. Dysmenorrhea and endometriosis in young women. *Yonago Acta Med.*, 2013 56(4), 81-84.

Harada, T; Momoeda, M; Terakawa, N; Taketani, Y; Hoshiai, H. Evaluation of a low-dose oral contraceptive pill for primary dysmenorrhea: a placebo-controlled, double-blind, randomized trial. *Fertil Steril*, 2011 95(6), 1928-1931.

Harrison, RF; Barry-Kinsella, C. Efficacy of medroxyprogesterone treatment in infertile women with endometriosis: a prospective, randomized, placebo-controlled study. *Fertil Steril*, 2000 74(1), 24-30.

Hornstein, MD; Hemmings, R; Yuzpe, AA; Heinrichs, WL. Use of nafarelin versus placebo after reductive laparoscopic surgery for endometriosis. *Fertil Steril*, 1997 68(5), 860-864.

Hornstein, MD; Surrey, ES; Weisberg, GW; Casino, LA. Leuprolide acetate depot and hormonal add-back in endometriosis: a 12-month study. Lupron Add-Back Study Group. *Obstet. Gynecol.*, 1998 91(1), 16-24.

Howard, FM. Endometriosis and mechanisms of pelvic pain. *J. Minim Invasive Gynecol.,* 2009 16(5), 540-550.

Jeon, GE; Cha, NH, Sok SR. Factors Influencing the Dysmenorrhea among Korean Adolescents in Middle School. *J. Phys. Ther. Sci.*, 2014 26(9), 1337-1343.

Kajitani, T; Maruyama, T; Asada, H; Uchida, H; Oda, H; Uchida, S; Miyazaky, K; Arase, T; Ono M; Yoshimura, Y. Possible involvment of nerve growth factor in dysmenorrhea and dyspareunia associated with endometriosis. *Endocr. J.,* 2013 60(10), 1155-1164.

Karck, U; Reister, F; Schäfer, W; Zahradnik, HP; Breckwoldt, M. PGE2 and PGF2 alpha release by human peritoneal macrophages in endometriosis. *Prostaglandins,* 1996 51(1), 49-60.

Koike, H; Egawa, H; Ohtsuka, T; Yamaguchi, M; Ikenoue, T; Mori, N. Correlation between dysmenorrheic severity and prostaglandin production in women with endometriosis. *Prostaglandins Leukot Essent Fatty Acids,* 1992 46(2), 133–137.

Koninckx, PR; Meuleman, C; Demeyere, S; Lesaffre, E; Cornillie, FJ. Suggestive evidence that pelvic endometriosis is a progressive disease, whereas deeply infiltrating endometriosis is associated with pelvic pain. *Fertil Steril*, 1991 55(4), 759-765.

Lockhat, FB; Emembolu, JO; Konje, JC. The evaluation of the effectiveness of an intrauterine-administered progestogen (levonorgestrel) in the symptomatic treatment of endometriosis and in the staging of the disease. *Hum. Reprod.*, 2004 19(1), 179-184.

Marjoribanks, J; Proctor, ML; Farquhar, C. Nonsteroidal anti-inflammatory drugs for primary dysmenorrhoea (Cochrane Review). *Cochrane Database of Systematic Reviews*, 2003 (4), CD001751.

Matsuzaki, S; Canis, M; Pouly, JL; Wattiez, A; Okamura, K , Mage G. Cyclooxygenase-2 expression in deep endometriosis and matched eutopic endometrium. *Fertil Sterill*, 2004 82(5), 1309-1315.

Mechsner, S; Kaiser, A; Kopf, A; Gericke, C; Ebert, A; Bartley, J. A pilot study to evaluate the clinical relevance of endometriosis-associated nerve fibers in peritoneal endometriotic lesions. *Fertil Steril*, 2009 92(6), 1856-1861.

Mechsner, S; Schawarz, J; Thode, J; Loddenkemper, C; Salomon, DS; Ebert, AD. Growth-associated protein 43- positive sensory nerve fibers accompanied by immature vessels are located in or near peritoneal endometriotic lesions. *Fertil Steril*, 2007 88(3), 581-587.

Mehedintu, C; Plotogea, M; Ionescu, S; Antonovici, M. Endometriosis still a challenge. *J. Med. Life*, 2014 7(3), 349-357.

Moran, C; Alcivia, JC; Garcia-Hernandez, E; Castro, J. Treatment of endometriosis with cyproterone acetate. Preliminary report. *Arch. Med. res,* 1996 27(4), 535-538.

Morotti, M; Sozzi, F; Remorgida, V; Venturini, PL; Ferrero, S. Dienogest in women with persistent endometriosis-related pelvic pain during norethisterone acetate treatment. *Eur. J. Obstet. Gynecol. Reprod. Biol.,* 2014b 183, 188-192.

Morotti, M; Vincent, K; Brawn, J; Zondervan, K T; Becker, C M. Peripheral changes in endometriosis-associated pain. *Human reproduction Update,* 2014a 20(5), 717-736.

Olavi, Y; Lasse V. Prostaglandin and endometriosis. *Acta Obset Gynecol scand Suppl,* 1983 113, 105-107.

Parazzini, F; Di Cintio, E; Chatenoud, L; Moroni, S; Ardovino, I; Struzziero, E; Falsett,i L; Bianchi, A; Bracco, G; Pellegrini, A; Bertulessi, C; Romanini, C; Zupi, E; Massobrio, M; Guidetti, D; Troiano, L; Beretta, P; Franchi, M. Estroprogestin vs. gonadotrophin agonists plus estroprogestin in the treatment of endometriosis-related pelvic pain: a randomized trial. Gruppo Italiano per lo Studio dell'Endometriosi. *Eur. J. Obstet. Gynecol. Reprod. Biol.*, 2000 88(1), 11-14.

Petraglia, F; Hornung, D; Seitz, C; Faustmann, T; Gerlinger, C; Luisi, S; Lazzeri, L; Strowitzki, T. Reduced pelvic pain in women with endometriosis: efficacy of long-term dienogest treatment. *Arch. Gynecol. Obstet.*, 2011 285(1), 157-173.

Petta, CA; Ferriani, RA; Abrao, MS; Hassan, D; Rosa, E; Silva, JC; Podgaec, S; Bahamondes, L. Randomized clinical trial of a levonorgestrel-releasing intrauterine system and a depot GnRH analogue for the treatment of chronic pelvic pain in women with endometriosis. *Hum. Reprod.*, 2005 20(7), 1993-1998.

Prentice, A; Deary, AJ; Goldbeck-Wood, S; Farquhar, C; Smith, SK. Gonadotrophin-releasing hormone analogues for pain associated with endometriosis. *Cochrane Database Syst. Rev.*, 2000 18(2), CD000346.

Propst, AM; Laufer MR. Endometriosis in adolescents. Incidence, diagnosis and treatment. *J. Reprod. Med.*, 1999 44(9), 751-758.

Razzi S; Luisi, S; Ferretti, C; Colanaci, F; Mazzini, M; Petraglia, F. Use of progestogen only preparation containing desogestrel in the treatment of recurrent pelvic pain after conservative surgery for endometriosis. *Eur. J. Obstet. Gynecol. Reprod. Biol.*, 2007 135(2), 188-190.

Remorgida, V; Abbamonte, HL; Ragni, N; Fulcheri, E; Ferrero, S. Letrozole and desogestrel-only contraceptive pill for the treatment of stage IV endometriosis. *Aust. N Z J Obstet. Gynaecol.*, 2007a 47(3), 222-225.

Remorgida, V; Abbamonte, HL; Ragni, N; Fulcheri, E; Ferrero, S. Letrozole and norethisterone acetate in rectovaginal endometriosis. *Fertil Steril,* 2007b 88(3), 724-726.

Scala, C; Leone, Roberti, Maggiore, U; Remorgida, V; Venturini, PL; Ferrero, S. Drug safety evaluation of desogestrel. *Expert Opin Drug Saf,* 2013 12(3), 433-444.

Schlaff, WD; Carson, SA; Luciano, A; Ross, D; Bergqvist, A. Subcutaneous injection of depot medroxyprogesterone acetate compared with leuprolide acetate in the treatment of endometriosis-associated pain. *Fertil Steril,* 2006 85(2), 314-325.

Selak, V; Farquhar, C; Prentice, A; Singla, A. Danazol for pelvic pain associated with endometriosis. *Cochrane Database Syst. Rev.*, 2007 17(4), CD000068.

Strowitzki, T; Faustmann, T; Gerlinger, C; Seitz, C. Dienogest in the treatment of endometriosis-associated pelvic pain: a 12-week, randomized, double-blind, placebo-controlled study. *Eur. J. Obstet. Gynecol. Reprod. Biol.*, 2010a 151(2), 193-198.

Strowitzki, T; Marr, J; Gerlinger, C; Faustmann, T; Seitz, C. Dienogest is as effective as leuprolide acetate in treating the painful symptoms of endometriosis: a 24-week, randomized, multicentre, open-label trial. *Hum. Reprod.*, 2010b 25(3), 633-641.

Sutton, CJ; Ewen, SP; Whitelaw, N; Haines, P. Prospective, randomized, double- blind, controlled trial of laser laparoscopy in the treatment of pelvic pain associated with minimal, mild, and moderate endometriosis. *Fertil Steril*, 1994 62(4), 696-700.

Telimaa, S; Puolakka, J; Ronnberg, L; Kauppila, A. Placebo-controlled comparison of danazol and high-dose medroxyprogesterone acetate in the treatment of endometriosis. *Gynecol. Endocrinol.*, 1987a 1(1), 13-23.

Telimaa, S; Ronnberg, L; Kauppila, A. Placebo-controlled comparison of danazol and high-dose medroxyprogesterone acetate in the treatment of endometriosis after conservative surgery. *Gynecol. Endocrinol.*, 1987b 1(4), 363-371.

Tokushige, N; Markham, R; Russel, P; Fraser, IS; Nerve fibers in peritoneal endometriosis. *Hum. Reprod.*, 2006 21(11), 3001-3007.

Tong, C; Conklin, D; Clyne, BB; Stanislaus, JD; Eisenach, JC. Uterine cervical afferents in thoracolumbar dorsal root ganglia express transient receptor potential vanilloid type 1 channel and calcitonin gene-related peptide, but not P2X3 receptor and somatostatin. *Anesthesiology,* 2006 104(4), 651-657.

Vercellini, P; De Giorgi, O; Oldani, S; Cortesi, I; Panazza, S; Crosignani, PG. Depot medroxyprogesterone acetate versus an oral contraceptive combined with very low-dose danazol for long-term treatment of pelvic pain associated with endometriosis. *Am. J. Obstet. Gynecol.*, 1996 175(2), 396-401.

Vercellini, P; Fedele, L; Pietropaolo, G; Frontino, G; Somigliana, E; Crosignani, PG. Progestogens for endometriosis: forward to the past. *Hum. Reprod. Update*, 2003a 9(4), 387-396.

Vercellini, P; Frontino, G; De Giorgi, O; Aimi, G; Zaina, B; Crosignani, PG. Comparison of a levonorgestrel-releasing intrauterine device versus expectant management after conservative surgery for symptomatic endometriosis: a pilot study. *Fertil Steril*, 2003b 80(2), 305-309.

Vercellini, P; Frontino, G; De Giorgi, O; Pietropaolo, G; Pasin, R; Crosignani, PG. Continuous use of an oral contraceptive for endometriosis-associated recurrent dysmenorrhea that does not respond to a cyclic pill regimen. *Fertil Steril*, 2003c 80(3),560-3.

Vercellini, P; Pietropaolo, G; De Giorgi, O; Pasin, R; Chiodini, A; Crosignani, PG. Treatment of symptomatic rectovaginal endometriosis with an estrogen-progestogen combination versus low-dose norethindrone acetate. *Fertil Steril*, 2005 84(5), 1375-1387.

Vignali, M; Bianchi, S; Candiani, M; Spadaccini, G; Oggioni, G; Busacca, MJ. Surgical treatment of deep endometriosis and risk of recurrence. *Minim Invasive Gynecol,* 2005 12(6), 508-513.

Walch, K; Unfried, G; Huber, J; Kurz, C; Van Trotsenburg, M; Pernicka, E; Wenzl, R. Implanon versus medroxyprogesterone acetate: effects on pain scores in patients with symptomatic endometriosis - a pilot study. *Contraception*, 2009 79(1), 29-34.

Weed, J C. Prostaglandins as related to endometriosis. *Clin. Obset. gynecol,* 1980 23(3), 895-900.

Whitehill, K; Yong, PJ, Williams, C. Clinical predictors of endometriosis in the infertility population: is there a better way to determine who needs a laparoscopy?. *J. Obstet. Gynaecol. Can*, 2012 34(6), 552-557.

William, EA; Colloins, WP; Clayton, SG. Studies in the involvement of prostaglandins in uterine symptomatology and pathology. *Br. J. Obset. Gynaecol.,* 1976 83(5), 337-341.

Wright, J; Lotfallah, H; Jones, K; Lovell, D. A randomized trial of excision versus ablation for mild endometriosis. *Fertil Steril*, 2005 83(6), 1830–1836.

Yeung, P, Jr; Tu, F; Bajzak, K; Lamvu, G; Guzovsky, O; Agnelli, R; Peavey, M; Winer, W; Albee, R; Sinervo, K. A pilot feasibility multicenter study of patients after excision of endometriosis. *JSLS,* 2013 17(1), 88-94.

Index

A

B

N

O

P